EATING 2.0

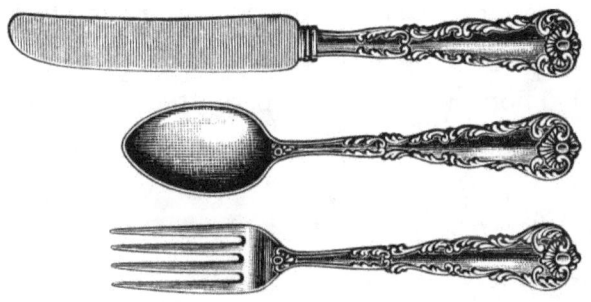

HOW TO EAT CONFIDENTLY IN
AN ULTRAPROCESSED WORLD

JEFF SIEGEL

JES Wellness

SOMERVILLE, MASSACHUSETTS

Jeff Siegel/JES Wellness
Somerville, Massachusetts
www.JeffSiegelWellness.com

Cover design by Steve Kuhn
Copy editing and book production by Stephanie Gunning

Special discounts are available on quantity purchases by corporations, associations, and others. For details, contact the author at the website above.

Eating 2.0/Jeff Siegel —first edition

Library of Congress Control Number 2025920478

ISBN 979-8-9891204-0-6 (paperback)
ISBN 979-8-9891204-2-0 (ebook epub)

DISCLAIMER

This book is for educational and informational purposes only. It is not medical advice, psychological counseling, or a substitute for professional diagnosis, treatment, or therapy. Reading this book or communicating with the author does not create a doctor-patient, dietitian-client, or therapist-client relationship. The author is not a licensed medical or mental health professional, and the ideas presented here should not replace guidance from a qualified healthcare provider.

If you have or suspect you may have an eating disorder or other medical condition, seek help from a licensed physician, registered dietitian, therapist, or other qualified health professional. Eating disorders can be life threatening. If you are in crisis or thinking about harming yourself, call or text a suicide-prevention helpline in your country. (In the United States, call or text 988.) If you think you may be experiencing a medical emergency, call emergency services immediately. (In the United States, call 911.)

Before making changes to your diet, physical activity, or treatment plan—especially if you are pregnant or breastfeeding, have a history of eating disorders or chronic illness, or take prescription medications—consult your doctor or another qualified clinician. Information in this book is general and may not apply to your circumstances; individual results will vary.

If this book references websites, products, or services, links are provided for information only. The author and publisher do not control and are not responsible for third-party content, and inclusion does not imply endorsement. The author and publisher disclaim any liability for injury, loss, or damage incurred directly or indirectly as a result of the use or misuse of the information contained in this book.

To Claire and Asher:

You are the ballast and sails of my boat. Without you, I'd be adrift, bailing water off the poop deck. This book exists because of your support. With all my love.

CONTENTS

PREFACE: *The Journey Begins*   *1*

INTRODUCTION: *Running Stone Age Software*   *13*
in a Food 2.0 World

Part I: The System Crash   27

CHAPTER 1: How Food 2.0 Hijacks What You Eat   29
Making Eating Irresistible, Effortless, Endless

CHAPTER 2: When Dinner Broke   63
The Three Disruptions That Forever Changed How You Eat

CHAPTER 3: The Three Dead-Ends   85
Why Diets and Intuition Can't Beat Food 2.0

Part II: The Internal Programming   99

CHAPTER 4: Revealing Your Code   101
The Four Keys to Food Freedom

CHAPTER 5: Your Survival Eater   123
The Relentless Guardian Who Fears Going Hungry

CHAPTER 6: Your Pleasure Eater   145
The Joy Seeker Who Wants Another Bite

CHAPTER 7: Your Social Eater   165
The Belonging Seeker Who Fears Being Left Out

CONTENTS

CHAPTER 8: Your Strategic Eater   189
The Ambitious Planner Who Wants Control

PART III: The Eating 2.0 Upgrade   215

CHAPTER 9: Inner Leadership   217
Taking the Seat at the Head of Your Own Table

CHAPTER 10: Outer Mastery   235
The Five Power Moves for Eating 2.0

CHAPTER 11: Making Peace with Food   251
Harmonizing the Desires That Pull You Apart

CHAPTER 12: Eating 2.0 In the Real World   267
Navigating Restaurants, Supermarkets, and Social Tables

EPILOGUE: The Dawn of Eating 3.0   299

ACKNOWLEDGMENTS   315

NOTES   321

RESOURCES: Continue Your Journey   333

ABOUT THE AUTHOR   335

PREFACE

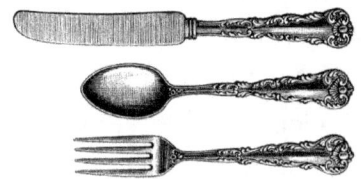

THE JOURNEY BEGINS

When I was diagnosed with anorexia nervosa at age fourteen—the eating disorder with the highest mortality rate of any psychiatric condition—I knew my relationship with food would color the rest of my life.[1] These were some of the hardest days and months I ever had. Despite saying that I wanted to live, I nearly starved myself to death. It got so bad that my parents pulled me out of high school and entered me into a residential hospital program. I was hesitant at first, but knew this was a necessary step to prevent me from falling further into the grips of mind-body warfare. In hindsight, the only reason I was able to pull myself from this dark place was because of my incredibly supportive family, a strong will to live, and extensive therapeutic resources.

Recovery wasn't a straight line. Health came gradually. Healing happened at the speed of trust between my present reality and my past compulsions. As I let go of one extreme or neurotic relationship with food, another would emerge—layers upon layers of psychological and emotional baggage coursed through my nervous system.

PREFACE

I made tremendous progress in eating normally (whatever that might be for a teenager), but I also dragged around a suitcase of fear and anxiety about my eating becoming dangerously out of balance again—The vestiges of the past were a heavy weight to carry. I knew deep in my heart that I wanted a balanced and peaceful relationship with food. I also knew the road ahead would be long and winding.

In my twenties, I adopted a mindset that was certainly better than extreme restriction: eating to fuel my body and support my workouts. However, this approach eventually became mechanical, stripping away emotions in favor of precalculated precision. I found myself eating as if I were a Ph.D. experiment in food science.

Do cashews raise my blood sugar more than almonds? Let me check my continuous glucose monitor.

Can I eat 4,000 calories today and still lower my body fat percentage tomorrow? Let's experiment and find out.

I would stand in supermarket aisles reading nutrition labels, comparing ingredients, and double-checking calorie math. I could recite nutrition facts verbatim: one serving of Cinnamon Toast Crunch: 3/4 cup, 130 calories, 3 grams fat, 25 grams carbs. While this made for fun party tricks, I knew the dark side of this obsession.

My goal was to understand every nuance of macronutrients and calories so I could control them, and in turn, control how my body looked and felt. Although it was enlightening to learn about nutrition, I felt a sense of defeat every time the math didn't add up. Eating perfectly was impossible. No matter how much I knew, my body played by its own rules.

Deep down, I knew this degree of control was unsustainable—a harsh truth every dieter eventually learns. The more I clung to an imagined version of how I "should" be eating, the more life threw food back in my face. I struggled to accept that eating for me will always be somewhat impulsive, somewhat intentional, and that's perfectly okay. My fear of losing control around food was actually a fear of losing love and my "thin privilege" —another way my mind had internalized fatphobic thoughts from diet culture. I had come a long way since my teenage years of restriction, but I still had a lot of healing to do to find a relationship with food that didn't take up so much mental bandwidth.

Caught Between Warring Camps

By my thirties, I was searching for a new approach to eating, but found myself caught between warring camps: the pro-diet side, promising health by controlling nutrients, and the anti-diet side, advocating for complete food freedom and body acceptance. Each camp seemed to have part of the truth, but neither offered a complete solution to our modern reality.

The diet side emphasized nutrition science, but overlooked the psychological damage of restriction and the relentless pursuit of thinness. The anti-diet side addressed the emotional toll of unrealistic beauty standards and body-size stigma, but often underemphasized the legitimate role of food's impact on one's health. Meanwhile, both sides largely ignored the complex sociocultural forces that make eating not only about personal preferences but also about class, gender, and privilege.

I felt lost in this siloed conversation. I didn't want to return to the black-and-white world of "good" and "bad" foods, but the alternative—pretending nutrients and calories don't matter— seemed equally inadequate in a world designed for mindless overconsumption. I couldn't find a coherent and integrated solution. The result was feeling stuck, struggling to live in the gray area between caring too much about what I ate and caring too little.

Questions like the following multiplied in my mind.

- *When does rejecting mainstream food culture become another form of disordered eating?*
- *How do I stay thoughtful about nutrition without becoming neurotic?*
- *Can I accept emotional eating as part of life without it becoming maladaptive?*
- *How do I eat responsibly in the moment while staying aligned with long-term goals?*
- *Is it possible to achieve the health and energy I want without specific goals or rigid eating rules?*

The Breakthrough:
Discovering Our Internal Multiplicity

Marc David doesn't know this, but he completely changed my life. While I was taking his course on dynamic eating psychology, in the middle of one of his lectures, he posed the question: Who decides what you eat?

He wasn't asking *what* I was eating. Not *how much* I was eating. Not *where, when,* or *with whom* I was eating. But *who?* Who was doing the choosing?

Marc was not referring to a parent or partner buying the food, setting the menu, or cooking for me and the other students. He was referring to the awareness behind the choice, the upstream consciousness, that make the decisions.

Who decided if I went for second helpings or turned down dessert?

Who was mindlessly shoveling morsels of food into my mouth while staring at my phone?

Who declined dressing but asked for extra protein?

Who was the character behind the scenes making the decisions? Was it me, Jeff? Or was someone else in charge?

These questions led me to the most significant discovery of my eating journey: "I" was not a single eater. I was manifold. "I" was a body trying to nourish itself *and* "I" was a collection of pleasure-seeking memories trying to recreate past satisfying bites. "I" was a set of health concepts trying to eat my way to perfect wellness *and* "I" was a social eater shaped by the people and the food choices they were making. "I" was a multiplicity of parts playing out their values, scripts, and needs.

The biggest realization was how all of this was happening beneath my awareness, which meant that "I" was not in as much control of my eating as I once thought—a scary thought for someone hell bent on controlling food.

At first, I didn't know what to do with the newfound awareness. Seeing myself as a collection of parts trying to get fed in different ways was helpful, but I still felt frustrated when one part of me said, "Let's eat," and another part said, "No way." I struggled to embrace messy emotions and contradictory drives that skirted structure and defied discipline. I needed new tools to reach into my shadows and work skillfully with this disharmony. Thankfully, that is exactly what I found when I was introduced to *Internal Family Systems* (IFS) *Therapy*.

IFS is an approach to individual psychotherapy developed by Richard Schwartz, Ph.D., that revolutionized the field of psychology by recognizing that we all have multiple "parts" within us—what I now refer to as the *Inner Eaters*—that represent distinct aspects of our personality. These parts develop organically to help us navigate life's challenges, but they can become distorted, extreme, or maladaptive over time. When parts become imbalanced or unreasonable, they can manifest as patterns of self-sabotage, compulsive behavior, or intrusive thoughts—exactly the things that make eating well a constant internal battle.

The key insight of IFS is that we can understand and work with these internal voices rather than pathologize them.

As I began applying IFS tools to eating—among them, self-leadership, unblending, and honoring my protector parts—I discovered newfound freedom in my relationship with food. I could be with my parts without being overwhelmed by them. I started naming these parts and tracking their appearances at mealtime. I found that there were four primary parts that consistently influenced my perception of food. I called these the Inner Eaters, and started using this framework to help manage the complexity I was feeling inside.

The language of Inner Eaters gave me just enough space to see new possibilities where I previously felt stifled. Each time I shifted from "What's wrong with me?" to "What makes sense about how my Inner Eaters organized themselves?" I created the foundation for healing. When I combined this approach with the nutritional discernment I developed as a result of my eating disorder, I finally felt like a breakthrough had occurred. I had the external skills to master modern food and the internal skills to harmonize the dynamic drives that tugged on my appetite. For the first time, I felt well-equipped to handle the vagaries and traps of twenty-first-century eating without getting lost in diet debates, hijacked by ultraprocessed food, or stuck in internal conflict. This was the beginning of Eating 2.0, and the foundation for everything I have included in this book.

The Theoretical Foundation:
Mapping Our Inner Eaters

The four Inner Eaters that I've identified follow developmental patterns explained by major psychological and sociological frameworks.

For one, the Inner Eaters in the Eating 2.0 system correspond remarkably well to Abraham Maslow's hierarchy of needs. The Survival Eater addresses basic physiological and safety needs—ensuring we have enough fuel to reproduce and avoid perceived threats. The Pleasure Eater corresponds with our need for variety and sensory satisfaction. The Social Eater fulfills our need for belonging and love through eating and cooking together. The Strategic Eater serves our esteem and achievement needs by using food to optimize performance and appearance. All of these parts ultimately serve our drive toward self-actualization—propelling us to become the people we're truly meant to be.

Even more fascinating, these Inner Eaters align with Spiral Dynamics, a developmental model devised by Clare W. Graves, Ph.D., that describes how human consciousness evolves from basic survival thinking through increasingly complex worldviews as life's conditions demand more sophisticated ways of operating. This development is evident both within individuals and societies at large. The interesting part is that development is rarely a straightforward one-way climb through the stages. (Hence, *spiral* dynamics, not *linear* dynamics.) You can move back to earlier stages when under stress, or climb to higher stages with adequate support. It's less about being "at" a particular stage and more about how you are relating to challenges in this moment, an idea that also seemed to be true with eating.

7

PREFACE

I found that the developmental stages of Spiral Dynamics perfectly captured the underlying value systems of each Inner Eater. If I were going to map each Inner Eater according to the stages of Spiral Dynamics, the Survival Eater would operate at an instinctive level, focusing on basic survival. The Pleasure Eater would embody the impulsive level, seeking immediate gratification. The Social Eater, which is rooted in the stage of order, would be emphasizing belonging and tradition. The Strategic Eater would represent the stage of achievement, focused on individual success and optimization. Each of these is an individual microcosm of the larger cultural worldviews that have evolved across human societies since the dawn of civilization.

The next stage in the Spiral Dynamics model is an egalitarian worldview, oriented toward social justice and environmental sustainability. This would be equivalent to an Ethical/Environmental Eater that considers the broader impact of our food choices on the planet. The intentions of this type of Inner Eater are evident in plant-based diets and businesses that prioritize environmental sustainability. I have gone back and forth as to whether ethical motivation for eating deserves its own chapter. For some, ethics or environmental concern might be a separate and significant part of their Inner Eater family. For others, it's just a flavor of the Strategic Eater, subsumed by more personal goals.

I imagine that as climate change puts increasing stress on our food systems, the Ethical/Environmental Eater will become more prominent—a fixture of people's consciousness as climate problems demand us to shift our thinking and eating to become more globally minded.

What excites me most is what emerges beyond an ethical eating stage. Spiral Dynamics and related Integral Theory posit a radical developmental leap that integrates and transcends all previous stages. The important part is that each previous stage—all the aforementioned Inner Eaters—represents a valid and necessary way of being in the world. Yet each one by itself is inadequate to handle the complexity of modern life. What is needed is an expansion of consciousness where you are no longer identified with any of the previous Inner Eaters. You need to be able to perceive all of them, understand their benefits, and acknowledge their limitations without judging any of them as right or wrong.

The magic of Eating 2.0 happens when you can access this expanded stage of consciousness. The path to get there is not by skipping stages or eliminating "lower" ones, but by integrating them all under the guidance of our most evolved awareness. A truly integrated eater can access their Survival Eater when genuinely needing nutrients, their Pleasure Eater when celebrating earthly joys, their Social Eater when connecting with others, and their Strategic Eater when pursuing health goals—all while being guided by deeper ethical wisdom and environmental concern. This is the evolution of eating that we are being called into, the eating upgrade we most desperately need.

The Larger Crisis

The work to heal our relationships with food feels particularly urgent right now. We're living through what many call a *polycrisis*— a period where our postmodern, globalized systems are unraveling and forces like climate change are threatening civilization as we know it. The old institutions, narratives, and ways of organizing reality that once provided stability and coherence are falling apart. Traditional food culture, family meal structures, and even our basic relationship with our bodies have

been disrupted by technological acceleration, social fragmentation, and cultural upheaval.

In this context, the question of how to eat becomes much more
than a personal health issue. It becomes a microcosm of the larger
challenge we all face: How do we create coherence and meaning
in a post-truth world that seems increasingly chaotic and disconnected? How do we integrate the best insights from different
traditions and disciplines without falling into rigid dogma or
relativistic confusion? Our current food system, which is built on
unconscious consumption, environmental destruction, and social
inequality, mirrors our internal fragmentation around eating.
Healing one heals the other.

The Journey Continues

For the last decade, I have coached hundreds of people, mostly
men, who were ready to end their war with food and eat
intentionally rather than habitually. I have been in the trenches of
frustration, poor health, and shame, with clients who were
struggling to find balance and were exhausted by "starting over"
each Monday. Everyone I have coached has had their unique
challenges with food, but underneath the surface issues was a
deeper challenge to love and respect themselves. Despite the
conditioning that taught them to control, berate, and hate their
body, they all shared the courage to grow into more comprehensive, peaceful, and purposeful humans. These were the seeds
we nurtured, and I cannot thank them enough for the privilege of
being their coach. It is because of their stories and lived experience that I have been able to form a system to bridge the artificial
divides between nutrition science and intuitive knowing, between
individual healing and cultural transformation, and between
ancient wisdom and modern innovation. This book is an outgrowth

of our work together and the many lessons (and missteps) we had along the way.

I wrote this book as an offering of hope, a way forward when all the other paths you've tried have led nowhere. I deeply believe you can feel at peace with food, not by silencing your desires, but by listening to them more deeply. At the very least, I encourage you to get to know your different eating parts because if there's one thing I've learned, it is this: Understanding who you are as an eater is not just helpful—it's essential. Without this internal awareness, you'll always make food choices based on inherited programming rather than your deeper wisdom.

The work of becoming a more integrated and empowered eater is the work of a lifetime (perhaps many lifetimes), one that extends far beyond mere survival into the realm of self-actualization. It calls us to remember that eating is not just a personal act, but a collective, ecological, embodied one. When we liberate ourselves from shame, confusion, and control over food, we help liberate others, too. When we evolve our eating habits from the inside out, we walk through the doorway toward wholeness, connection, and becoming more fully ourselves. And in a world where the old maps no longer match the territory, we need new ways of eating consciously that honor the full complexity of being human in the twenty-first century.

Even in the face of global disorder and inner chaos, you can choose care, joy, and the steady discipline of inner leadership. When you shift your self-concept and expand the purpose of eating itself, your "hunger" may grow. Do not be alarmed. This doesn't mean you're about to eat everything in sight. But it does mean that eating itself will become an act of loving yourself and loving the world, for the two are intimately intertwined. After all, what is eating if not the magical nexus that connects all life in a marvelous web of transformation?

A Note on Privilege and Perspective

I'm writing this book as a white, cisgender, heterosexual, Jewish American man raised in a professional, educated household in Philadelphia. I grew up with enough to eat, access to excellent healthcare and education, and a strong support system— advantages that shaped my path and perspective. I also recognize that not everyone has these resources or was raised in an upper-middle-class American food culture. These social factors and identity locations significantly influence my perspective, so I want to acknowledge them upfront as personal biases and take responsibility for the blind spots they may create.

While this book assumes a large degree of individual choice when it comes to the food you eat, I recognize food is not just a personal issue about what you most want to eat; it's shaped by systems: economic, cultural, and historical. For many, eating well is not merely about selecting the best food in the grocery store or off the menu, but about navigating inequality, scarcity, stress, and basic survival. I don't pretend to speak for every experience, but I've written this book with deep respect for everyone who has struggled with food, body, and eating in some way, shape, or form. I aim to offer tools that help you reclaim agency—whether you're battling inner critics, outer constraints, or both—and to honor the strength it takes to pursue healing in a world that doesn't always make it easy to eat with awareness and intention.

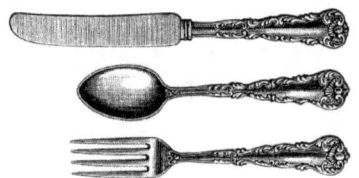

RUNNING STONE AGE SOFTWARE
IN A FOOD 2.0 WORLD

"We want a burst in the beginning," the flavor scientist explained. "And maybe a finish that doesn't linger too much—so you want more of it."

"So you don't want it to linger?" the CBS reporter asked, puzzled.

"No, because if it lingers, you're not going to eat more of it."

"It's got to be a quick fix," the reporter quipped with a knowing smile.

Manipulating the aftertaste was only the beginning. The following sentence was delivered like a confession.

"And then have more." The scientist paused before continuing, "And then have more. One bite is never enough."

"But that suggests something else . . . which is called *addiction*," said the reporter.

"Exactly," said the flavorist.

"You're trying to create an addictive taste?"

INTRODUCTION

"That's a good word—something that they want to go back for *again and again.*"[1]

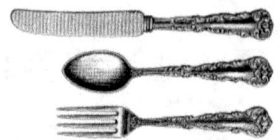

IF YOU'VE EVER felt like food is getting the best of you, or you give into temptations too easily, it's not because you're weak. It's because the system is rigged. The conversation above is not a fabricated story. It is the actual transcript from a 2011 episode of *60 Minutes* featuring an interview with veteran journalist Morley Safer.

The food scientist being interviewed worked for Givaudan, the largest flavoring company in the world. With over $7 billion in revenue, to the present day Givaudan creates customized flavors for many of the world's largest food brands. These flavors aren't just simple lemon and lime; they're precisely engineered formulas designed to keep you eating. The company sells these secret blends under strict confidentiality agreements, ensuring that the magic behind their addictive appeal remains undisclosed. And guess what? You've probably tasted their creations more times than you think.

That bag of chips dusted with a "proprietary seasoning," that caramel macchiato with just the right balance of sweetness and bitterness, that energy bar that somehow tastes like dessert but is marketed as "healthy," all might be the work of Givaudan's flavor architects, crafting food that tricks your brain into craving more. As the flavor scientist so blatantly spelled out, these foods are designed to hit your palate just hard enough to make you want more, but never enough to satisfy you fully.

Welcome to Food 2.0, an entirely new era of eating that is engineered to hijack your appetite, stimulate your desire, and exploit your biological vulnerabilities. This isn't food as your great-grandparents knew it. This is engineered eating.

The Unfair Fight We're In

Find it. Kill it. Grow it. Eat it. Survive. Repeat. These were the rules of eating for hundreds of thousands of years. Sugar was rare, found mainly in seasonal fruit. Fat was precious, available only after a successful hunt. Salt was so valuable that Roman soldiers were paid in it (hence the word *salary*). In this environment of scarcity, we developed the following predilections.

- Crave sweet things (quick energy)
- Seek out fatty foods (vital for later)
- Value salt (gather essential minerals)
- Eat opportunistically (maximize survival)
- Store excess energy (protect against famine)

These instincts served us well, until they didn't. In just the past few generations, food has morphed into what I call Food 2.0, a world of eating engineered for irresistible taste and corporate profit. Four aspects of Food 2.0 set it apart from the food our great-grandparents ate.

- **It tastes too good to say no.** Its hallmarks are hyper-palatable flavors, soft textures, and constant availability.

- **It is engineered at the molecular level.** Refined grains, oils, sugars, and additives hijack the brain's reward system.

- **It thrives in snack culture.** Meals give way to grazing, reheating, and distracted screen-side eating, all wrapped in health halos and endless marketing.

- **It depends on global industrial systems.** Monocrops, factory farming, aggressive product placement, and political lobbying make Food 2.0 omnipresent and cheap.

Taken together, Food 2.0 is an era of superabundance unlike anything planet Earth has ever seen, and the products it spits out are as evolutionarily novel as the first atom bomb—powerful, dazzling, and impossible to put back in the box.

In this system:

- Sugar isn't just in fruit anymore; it's in most packaged foods and concentrated many times beyond what you might find in nature.

- Fat isn't rare; it's everywhere—mainly in the form of industrially extracted seed oils.

- Salt isn't precious; it's commonplace, often hiding where you'd least expect it. (For instance, a Mexicali Salad from the Cheesecake Factory has a whopping 3,040 milligrams of sodium; that's over thirteen of those little salt packets you can get at a fast-food restaurant and 132 percent of the recommended daily limit.[2])

- Food isn't scarce. We're surrounded by cheap, abundant calories.

- Excess energy storage is no longer helpful insurance. It's now a global health crisis.

Here's the problem: Our eating instincts evolved for a Stone Age world where food was scarce, seasonal, and required significant effort to acquire. That world no longer exists.[3]

The Overdue Upgrade

Imagine trying to run the latest software on a computer from 1995. It crashes, freezes, and can't keep up. That's exactly what's happening when your ancient neurological wiring encounters the Food 2.0 environment. It glitches every time you eat what is considered normal and see the scale constantly creeping higher. It crashes when you're told, "Listen to your body," but you're busy staring at a screen and forget you even have a body. It freezes each time you are advised, "Eat only when you're hungry," but when are you *not* hungry?

No wonder eating well feels impossible. We're dealing with Frankenfoods, fractured culture, and broken systems that we try to patch with hacks such as:

- Cutting back on sugars.
- Trying intermittent fasting.
- Counting calories.
- Using GLP-1 drugs.
- Ditching the carbs or fats or seed oils or lectins or what have you.
- Opting for an "Every food fits" or "Everything will kill you somehow" attitude and losing all discernment.

When we try any of these fixes, it feels like an improvement for a while. However, the core issue remains: We're still relying on Stone Age software in a Food 2.0 world. Patchwork hacks won't cut it.

We're fighting a war we didn't sign up for against an enemy we can barely see and with weapons we don't understand. On one side, there's a multitrillion-dollar food industry armed with Givaudan engineers marketing products that are irresistible, effortless, and endless. On the other side is us, armed just with our willpower and good intentions.

Can you guess who's winning?

The evidence is everywhere. Despite having access to more nutritional information than any generation in history, rates of obesity, diabetes, and eating disorders in our society continue to climb. And despite collectively spending billions on diets, supplements, and wellness programs, most of us feel more confused and conflicted about food than ever before.

The solution isn't another diet. It is a complete eating upgrade.

The Rise of the Inner Eaters

Here's what I discovered after years of struggling with my own relationship with food, working with hundreds of clients, and studying the intersection of neuroscience, psychology, and nutrition: You don't have one relationship with food. You have several.

In fact, you have multiple "selves" that approach food for different reasons—a concept inspired by Internal Family Systems therapy, which helped bring the idea of "parts work" into the mainstream. These selves, which I call your Inner Eaters, line up with four fundamental purposes for eating.

Your reasons for eating include:

- **Survival**: to meet your body's basic needs.
- **Pleasure**: because food tastes good and feels good.

- **Social connection**: because as social mammals, sharing food has always meant safety.
- **Strategic goals**: to serve your long-term health, fitness, or appearance.

The problem? You are not any of these Inner Eaters. You are something bigger—someone who can observe and guide all these different parts of yourself. In Internal Family Systems, this observing part is called the *Self*. In *Eating 2.0*, we call it your conscious inner leader: the version of you that can rise above the chatter, hold each Inner Eater with wisdom and compassion, and understand what each needs without being hijacked by any single voice.

The issue is that it's hard to access your conscious leadership when you've spent a lifetime identifying with one or more of your Inner Eaters. That's why you can finish lunch swearing you're "done" for the day, only to find yourself elbow deep in a bag of popcorn at 3 PM. One part of you wants comfort. Another wants discipline. Another wants to be included. Another just wants to avoid hunger. You're constantly switching drivers without even realizing it.

Let me show you what I mean.

It's 3 PM on a Tuesday. You're standing in your kitchen, tired from attending back-to-back meetings, staring into the pantry. There's a bag of chips inside it, calling your name.

One part of you—let's call it your **Survival Eater**—sees the chips and thinks, *I'm depleted. I need energy now. I don't know when I'll eat again with this crazy schedule.*

Another part of you—your **Strategic Eater**—sees the same chips and raises a red flag. *Those chips are canola oil disguised as crunch. I'm going to feel crummy if I eat them. Plus, I have a nice dinner planned. Let's not ruin that.*

19

Same moment. Same food. Two completely different Inner Eaters. Two completely different reactions.

Most people experience this type of moment as an internal conflict: a battle between so-called "good" and "bad" impulses. But nothing is wrong with you. These are just different parts of you, each trying to take care of something important. Your Survival Eater isn't trying to sabotage you; it's trying to keep you alive. Your Strategic Eater isn't trying to punish you; it's trying to help you achieve your lofty goals.

Alongside them, you also have a **Pleasure Eater** that seeks joy and comfort and a **Social Eater** that craves connection and belonging. In a healthy food environment, these four Inner Eaters work together beautifully. But Food 2.0 has turned them against each other. Food 2.0 triggers your Survival Eater with artificial scarcity and chronically stressed lifestyles. It hijacks your Pleasure Eater with foods engineered to be more rewarding than anything found in nature. It manipulates your Social Eater with cultural messaging about what "good" people eat. And it overwhelms your Strategic Eater with conflicting information and impossible standards. It's like asking your brain for a simple dinner suggestion and getting a 300-comment group chat instead. It's too much.

The Promise of Eating 2.0

Eating 2.0 is not a new diet, but a radical upgrade to your entire eating operating system. The purpose of Eating 2.0 is not to conquer hunger or follow perfect rules. The purpose is to grow, adapt, and consciously lead yourself through the engineered world of Food 2.0.

Eating 2.0 begins by reclaiming your power, leading your Inner Eaters from the siren song of Food 2.0 back to a place of balance. When you learn to notice their drives without ignoring hunger, avoiding pleasure, resisting social meals, or over optimizing, you'll stop being pushed around by their unconscious agendas. You can start making conscious choices that build trust in yourself, knowing that you are not broken, and no matter what happens, you can return to your position as the conscious leader of your eating family.

Five Reasons This Works When Everything Else Fails

Eating 2.0 does not try to resolve the multilayered, emotionally charged complexity of modern eating. Rather, it teaches a *way of being* that is relational and responsive to the complex demands on our appetite. This new approach will benefit you for the following five specific reasons.

REASON 1. IT ENDS THE INTERNAL WAR

Most dietary approaches pit you against your cravings, impulses, or past behaviors. For instance, they may tell you to ignore your hunger (suppressing your Survival Eater), avoid pleasurable foods (shaming your Pleasure Eater), resist dining out (isolating your Social Eater), or follow rigid rules (turning your Strategic Eater into a tyrant). This never works because it forces you to suppress parts of yourself in a game of compliance, control, and perfectionism. When you demonize your Inner Eaters, they fight back—internal war breeds backlash.

By contrast, Eating 2.0 invites you to get curious about your Inner Eaters. It helps you map the web of relationships and tensions of your internal parts rather than silence them. And when you release rigid control that makes you feel wrong about some

21

aspect of yourself, you can build internal peace that creates the foundation for real, lasting transformation.

REASON 2. IT BUILDS SELF-COMPASSION AND ACCEPTANCE OF WHO YOU ARE

Every Inner Eater developed for a reason. When you understand their positive intentions, shame can give way to compassion. For example, you will learn to give space for your Strategic Eater's concern for sustainability without shaming your Survival Eater's need for ease. Both Inner Eaters have something valuable to offer, even if it's only been expressed poorly until now. Once you view your parts with kindness, you will be able to work with their natural tensions rather than collapsing into harsh self-criticism on occasions when you didn't act the way you wanted.

REASON 3. IT HONORS CONTEXT AND TRADEOFFS

There is no one-size-fits-all diet. There is only the dynamic interaction between your Inner Eaters and the food environment you inhabit. In other words, eating well is always relational, contextual, and highly individual. Eating habits that work in one culture, family, or body type may not be effective in another. This does not mean all foods are equally nutritious, but it does mean that a single choice of what, when, or how much to eat will require tradeoffs between your Inner Eaters. Recognizing that you can't always predict the long-term impacts of any single choice frees you from the grip of perfectionism and enables you to respond with humility to what is true right now.

REASON 4. IT CREATES SUSTAINABLE, SYSTEM-LEVEL TRANSFORMATION

When you listen to all your Inner Eaters, not just the loudest one, you can shift the system, not just surface symptoms. Working at this level will create changes in your thinking and behavior that support your whole self. Rather than bulldozing one goal over every other need, you create space for negotiation and integration—a relationship with food that evolves with you instead of against you.

REASON 5. IT TRANSFORMS EATING INTO A PATH FOR SELF-ACTUALIZATION

Cravings aren't failures; they're signals. A late-night snack might be your Pleasure Eater calling for comfort or your Social Eater needing connection. Eating 2.0 sees every bite as data. Every meal is an opportunity for personal growth and development. When eating becomes an awareness practice, you will become less reactive, not because you're perfectly disciplined, but because you're attuned to the deeper messages behind your hunger. In turn, this will open a door in you for self-actualization and self-transcendence to occur as you are learning to integrate your needs, your values, and your relationships through the act of eating itself.

How This Book Is Structured: Your Upgrade Path

This book follows a sequential approach that facilitates trans-formation. Each of the three parts builds on the previous one to help you become the conscious leader of your eating.

Part One, "The System Crash." The book starts with an analysis of what's happening around us. Here, you'll discover how our abundant food environment has been engineered to override our natural instincts, why modern life makes balanced eating nearly impossible, and why the solutions you've tried before were doomed from the start. Understanding these external forces isn't about blame or giving up; it's about wise discernment. You can't effectively lead your Inner Eaters without first understanding how they've been manipulated by Food 2.0.

Part Two, "The Internal Programming," Once you understand the external forces at play, we'll examine your internal operating system. You'll learn the CARE framework: how curiosity, appreciation, responsibility, and exploration will transform your hunger and relationship with food. You'll meet your four Inner Eaters—the fundamental "code" that runs the "software" of your eating decisions. You'll get detailed portraits of each Inner Eater: its evolutionary origins, its gifts and shadows, and how to work with it skillfully in modern life.

Part Three, "The Eating 2.0 Upgrade." In the book's final part, you'll be taught to integrate your external awareness with your internal wisdom to create a complete eating system that works in the modern world. You'll learn to lead your Inner Eaters through challenging situations, build supportive environments, and maintain dynamic harmony even when the world is pulling your appetite in every possible direction.

Throughout this book, you'll find many stories: some drawn from my own life, others inspired by friends, clients, and patterns I've witnessed again and again in my work. To protect privacy, I've changed names and details, and in some cases, combined elements from multiple people into fictional characters.

Many of these vignettes lean toward the extreme. That's intentional. When the gifts and blind spots of your Inner Eaters are exaggerated, they're easier to recognize. At the same time, I want to be clear: These examples are not meant to pathologize everyday eating or depict disordered eating in a clinical sense. They're teaching tools, designed to help you see your own patterns more clearly.

By the time you have finished this book, you'll be able to walk into any food situation and make choices that serve your whole life, not just your immediate cravings. You'll be empowered to eat without guilt, second-guessing yourself, or exhausting internal debates. Ultimately, you'll feel a sense of pride—and relief—that you can navigate the world of Food 2.0 without feeling like a victim of forces beyond your control.

What This Means for Your Daily Life

Imagine walking into the same kitchen we were discussing a few pages ago at 3 PM on a Tuesday, and instead of experiencing internal chaos or mindless munching, you simply feel curious. You notice your Survival Eater panicking about the hours since lunch and three meetings ahead with no break. You see your Strategic Eater worried about falling back into haphazard patterns.

Instead of reacting impulsively, you ask yourself: *How can I honor both needs?* Maybe those leftover roasted sweet potatoes with some nuts are a good starting place.

Same kitchen. Similar situation. Completely different experience.

No guilt. No confusion. No internal warfare. Just conscious leadership of your Inner Eater "family."

This is what becomes possible after you upgrade to Eating 2.0. This is what happens when you stop allowing yourself to be pushed around by unconscious forces and start to listen, understand, and coordinate your Inner Eaters toward a shared vision of well-being.

25

INTRODUCTION

The Responsibility for What You Eat Is Yours

You didn't choose to inherit Stone Age software or be born into a Food 2.0 world designed to exploit you. Nonetheless, you are 100 percent responsible for upgrading your eating habits.

No one else can develop your awareness, lead your Inner Eaters, or navigate Food 2.0 on your behalf. That's your work to do—and it may be the most essential upgrade you'll ever make.

If you're ready to stop forcing food to fit your outdated instincts and start leading yourself with Eating 2.0, turn the page. Let's begin.

PART I
THE SYSTEM CRASH

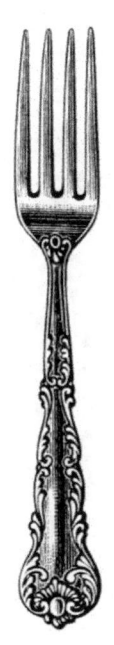

ONE

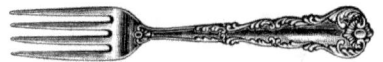

HOW FOOD 2.0 HIJACKS WHAT YOU EAT

MAKING EATING IRRESISTIBLE, EFFORTLESS, ENDLESS

"If sugar is the methamphetamine of processed food ingredients, with its high-speed, blunt assault on our brains, then fat is the opiate, a smooth operator whose effects are less obvious but no less powerful."

MICHAEL MOSS

The restaurant was bustling with energy, the clatter of plates and chatter filling the air.

Eight teenagers slid into their high-top seats, one by one. A server handed them a menu with over thirty options and a sealed envelope to be opened only after they had placed their orders. After a moment of reading over the menu, each teen made their choice and continued as usual.

As they sat comfortably waiting for their meals, the server told them they could open their sealed envelopes. They unfolded a piece of paper that read in bold text: "Triple-Dipped Chicken." They stared at the paper in disbelief.

Not just one person, but all eight had ordered the triple-dipped chicken. How did this happen?

These teens had been set up using the same techniques that big food companies use to craft and manipulate desire. These youngsters were bombarded with advertisements specifically for triple-dipped chicken before their restaurant visit. Images of crispy fried chicken showed up on flyers posted near their homes and on consoles in the taxi cabs that had brought them to the restaurant. The researchers even hired Instagram influencers to take videos of themselves eating huge bites of . . . you guessed it . . . triple-dipped chicken.[1]

After the fact, the teens were told how they had been manipulated. They claimed not to notice the ads, but the marketing had worked its magic. Every single teen zeroed in on the same exact food from a long list of other options. It was more than just a coincidence. It was Food 2.0 in action.

What Is Food 2.0?

Food 2.0 is my term for the modern food system that thrives on engineered consumption. It encompasses both the products—hyperpalatable, calorically dense, ultraprocessed foods—and the broader forces that normalize their presence in daily life, such as around-the-clock snacking, on-demand food delivery, billion-dollar marketing campaigns, and global systems that make eating effortless and endless. Unlike food grown close to home, prepared by hand, and lacking conspicuous labels or health claims, Food 2.0 is formulated, lab-optimized, and designed to capture your appetite and wallet.

Consider triple-dipped chicken. Triple dipping is a method of coating chicken pieces by dipping them twice into a dry flour mixture and once into a wet batter (like egg or beer batter) to create an extra-crispy, thicker crust when fried. This multilayered coating retains seasoning well, enabling food manufacturers to add salt, thickeners, artificial flavors, and other ingredients to enhance properties such as texture and mouthfeel. When you take this already alluring fried chicken and slather a sugary, sticky sauce on top, you've got an intensely rewarding, calorically dense, chemically altered food that is nearly impossible to resist.[2]

Next, consider how the teens in this experiment were manipulated by Food 2.0 marketing. It's no secret that the fast-food and beverage industries spend billions on marketing and product placement to ensure your cravings are constantly provoked. In fact, many of the world's largest food manufacturers have hired former tobacco executives who perfected addiction strategies to hook people on cigarettes. Philip Morris, one of the largest tobacco companies, actually owned Kraft Foods for decades, where it applied the same playbook that made its cigarettes irresistible to smokers to making macaroni and cheese, Oreos, and Velveeta equally hard for consumers to resist.[3]

Modern eating has left the realms of hunger and health, venturing boldly into manufactured desire. The result is that we continue to eat more, buy more, and consume more, until we experience a stomachache or have polished off the last crumbs lingering at the bottom of the container. There's no secret conspiracy driving us to become "snackaholics." It's blatant biochemical and marketing manipulation.

What's Changed with Food 2.0?
A Tale of Three Meals

The challenge today is that you might not even notice or realize how much you've already been swayed by the invisible hand of Food 2.0. You might think you're eating the same foods your grandparents did, just in more convenient packaging. You're not.

Let's take a chicken dinner—one from 1949 and one from today—and compare what's really on the plate.

CHICKEN DINNER (1949)

A home-cooked meal made from whole ingredients in 1949 included:

- A freshly butchered chicken, raised on a pasture where it was free to forage.
- Hand-peeled potatoes boiled and mashed with real butter and whole milk.
- Seasonal vegetables grown locally without synthetic pesticides or genetic modification.
- A slice of homemade bread made from flour, water, yeast, and salt.

This meal wasn't designed to manipulate your senses. It was simply food. It took time to prepare. If you left it out, it would quickly spoil. If certain ingredients weren't seasonally available, you were out of luck. As my brother would say, "You get what you get and don't get upset."

In a world without globalized supply chains and endless abundance, nobody got to be choosy about what was for dinner.

CHICKEN DINNER (TODAY)

A modern version of the same meal includes:

- A factory-farmed chicken pumped with antibiotics, bred for rapid weight gain, and fed a diet of corn and soy to maximize its size, possibly frozen and then thawed.

- Instant mashed potatoes made from dehydrated potato flakes containing artificial flavorings and emulsifiers to enhance their texture.

- Greenhouse vegetables grown abroad, which are coated in pesticides and have been shipped thousands of miles before reaching your supermarket.

- Factory-made bread loaded with high-fructose corn syrup, dough conditioners, and shelf stabilizers to extend its lifespan.

To the untrained eye, these two meals might look identical. However, the reality is that they couldn't be more different. The 1949 meal was unfeigned food. The modern meal is a product engineered for portability, palatability, and profit.

A CONTEMPORARY ULTRAPROCESSED CHICKEN DINNER

Let's examine the label for a specific chicken dinner found in the freezer section of most major supermarkets in the United States: Stouffer's Baked Chicken Frozen Meal. When you look at the ingredient list, you may wonder why chicken with gravy and mashed potatoes requires nearly fifty ingredients. The chicken fillets inside the package are described as:

COOKED CHICKEN BREAST FILLETS (CHICKEN BREAST FILLETS, WATER, BROWN SUGAR, MODIFIED RICE STARCH, CANOLA OIL, CHICKEN FLAVOR [DRIED CHICKEN BROTH, CHICKEN POWDER, FLAVOR, SALT], SODIUM PHOSPHATES, CARRAGEENAN, SALT, WHITE PEPPER, PAPRIKA).

This product begins with a chicken breast, a hit of sugar, and a significant amount of food science behind the scenes. Ingredients such as modified rice starch, sodium phosphates, and carrageenan are added to the food to maintain stability, improve mouthfeel, alter texture, and make the product more appealing.

Rather than relying on real chicken for flavor, this blend of seasonings uses dried chicken broth, chicken powder, and the general term *flavor*, which is vague and could encompass a wide range of artificial or chemical additives. The company's goal is to deliver chicken taste quickly and cheaply. The question is, why doesn't the chicken itself provide that flavor?

The laundry list of flavoring agents, emulsifiers, and preservatives goes on. While these ingredients may prevent spoilage, they also are associated with serious health concerns.

- Emulsifiers such as carrageenan in the Stouffer's chicken dinner, and others like carboxymethylcellulose or polysorbate 80 can disrupt our gut microbiomes, leading to inflammation and metabolic disturbances.[4]

- Artificial sweeteners, including aspartame and sucralose, have been linked to alterations in glucose metabolism and increased risk of type 2 diabetes.[5]

- Nitrates and nitrites, commonly used in processed meats, can form carcinogenic compounds in the body, elevating the risk of colorectal cancer.[6]

- Packaging contaminants like bisphenol A (BPA) and phthalates can leach into food, acting as endocrine disruptors and potentially contributing to obesity and reproductive issues.[7]

While each of these substances poses risks, the cumulative effect of these additives, combined with high levels of sugar, salt, and unhealthy fats, contributes to the overall health hazards associated with ultraprocessed foods.

Stouffer's Baked Chicken Frozen Meal is the perfect example of a fatty, salty, synthetically made meal. It may lure your calorie consciousness into complicity at only 260 calories per package, but that misses the point. You're buying into an entire system that profits from delivering an artificially contrived eating experience with minimal nutrients at minimal cost.

The harm of Food 2.0 emerges not from a single meal, but from the synergy: the proprietary recipe that highjacks your tastebuds, the scale of production that makes it ubiquitous, the marketing strategy that makes it alluring, and the dietary patterns that result from all of these forces combined. Asking which specific part of Food 2.0 is to blame—the additives or advertisements, the sugar or the seductive messaging—is like asking which snowflake caused an avalanche.[8] When you consider how all of these factors work together to scramble the sense-making of your Inner Eaters, the problem becomes clear.

The Triple Threat:
How Food 2.0 Hijacks our Inner Eaters

Modern food isn't just different from what our grandparents ate, it's engineered using three specific strategies to keep us eating more.

Hijack 1. Make it irresistible. Food 2.0 intentionally utilizes bliss points, precise combinations of sugar, salt, and fat, to activate our brain's reward centers in a manner similar to addictive drugs.

Hijack 2. Make it effortless. Ultraprocessed foods are pre-chewed, softened, and stripped of fiber so you can consume massive calories without your body registering fullness.

Hijack 3. Make it endless. Supersized portions, shelf-stable ingredients, and infinite variety ensure you never run out of options to choose from or hit natural stopping points when eating.

Let's see how each of these strategies targets your Inner Eaters.

Hijack 1. Make It Irresistible

My toddler son loves going to Costco. The massive aisles stacked high with endless towers of goods feel like an adventure, a kingdom of possibility for a two-year-old. But his favorite part? The free samples.

He sits eagerly in the cart, scanning the floor like a hawk. He tenses with excitement the moment he spots a sample station setting up. We make our way over, and as soon as he gets his bite-sized treasure, he pops it into his mouth with pure delight. But before he's even finished chewing, his hands are already reaching out again. "More," he demands. "I want more!"

At first, it's endearing. A simple moment of childhood joy. But this isn't how he reacts when I offer him an apple or a handful of baby carrots. He loves fruit, but it doesn't send him into a frenzy. This response is indicative that my son's chasing a high.

The difference? The food we are sampling wasn't picked from a tree or pulled from the soil. It was something designed and engineered for maximum bliss. Perfectly crispy. Satisfyingly crunchy. Just enough salt to stimulate his taste buds, enough fat to coat his tongue in pleasure, and enough umami to make every bite feel deeply rewarding.

When I saw this happen the first time, I realized his reaction to the food sample wasn't just about hunger or even about preference, it was about chemistry. His brain was lighting up in ways nature never intended, *wired to crave more* before he swallowed the first bite.

THE SCIENCE OF BLISS POINTS, HYPERPALATABILITY, AND FOOD ADDICTION

The multibillion-dollar food industry isn't in the business of nourishment. It's in the business of cravings. Imagine the perfect bite of food—not too salty, not too sweet, just enough fat. It hits all the right notes before fading quickly. The result is that you immediately want another bite. This is called the *bliss point*, a term coined by food scientist Howard Moskowitz to describe the precise combination of sugar, fat, and salt that maximizes pleasure and minimizes satiety.

The bliss point isn't guesswork. It's science. Decades of research have revealed that the perfect ratio of sugar, fat, and salt can light up our brain's reward centers, creating a pleasure loop eerily similar to addictive drugs. In fact, food manufacturers spend millions tweaking these ratios.

The outcome? Foods that taste so good they short-circuit our ability to stop eating. You might think, *I don't eat chips, fast food, or junk food, so this doesn't apply to me.* But hyperpalatability isn't just about neon-colored snack foods. Many modern foods are designed with the bliss point in mind.

Consider something as simple as rotisserie chicken, a staple in my household. At first glance, it seems like a wholesome, high-protein food. But supermarket versions are often injected with sugar, salt, and flavor-enhancing solutions to keep them juicy and irresistibly tasty. Ingredients like yeast extract, hydrolyzed vegetable protein, or soy protein isolate may seem odd to add to chicken, but they are flavor enhancers designed to improve savory notes. That's why a fresh rotisserie chicken from the store may disappear far quicker than a plain chicken you make at home. One is doctored up; the other is not.

Or take roasted nuts, a nutritious snack in moderation. But coat them in honey, sea salt, or chili-lime seasoning, and suddenly, they go from satisfying to addictive. Their salty-sweet-fatty profile lights up your tastebuds, making it easy to mindlessly eat half a bag before you even realize it. I've done this so many times that you think I would've learned my lesson. I never do.

That "healthy" breakfast granola might seem full of wholesome nuts and seeds. But when you look closer, you might find evaporated cane juice, fruit juice concentrate, barley malt, rice syrup, agave nectar—all types of sugar. In fact, sugar hides on ingredient lists under more than sixty different names. Companies may use multiple sugar sources clustered together to prevent sugar from appearing as the first ingredient. It's one sweet coverup.

Perhaps the most fascinating and potentially problematic form of bliss point engineering exists in diet foods and artificial sweeteners. These products represent a unique type of sensory manipulation. They're designed to deliver the same hyper-palatable experience while technically containing fewer calories.

When you consume a diet soda or artificially sweetened yogurt, your taste buds detect intense sweetness and send signals to your brain and digestive system, preparing them for an incoming sugar load. Your pancreas releases insulin, your brain anticipates the reward of calories, and your digestive system prepares for energy processing, but the expected calories never arrive.

This creates a type of metabolic "confusion," where the normal relationship between sweet taste and caloric content becomes decoupled. Studies suggest this disconnection may actually increase cravings and hunger as your body seeks the calories it was promised but never received.[9] Over time, this can desensitize your natural sweetness perception, making naturally sweet foods like fruit seem less satisfying.

The diet product paradox represents how sophisticated food engineering can create unintended consequences, disrupting the complex hormonal signaling systems that regulate appetite and fundamentally changing how your body perceives reward.

LAYERING SENSORY CONTRAST: MULTIDIMENSIONAL DELICIOUSNESS

Consider the humble Brussels sprout. This perfectly healthy vegetable has undergone a dramatic makeover. For years, it was steamed with a dash of salt or butter. It was filling, fibrous, and maybe not anyone's favorite vegetable, but a nice accompaniment to a meal.

In the 1990s, chefs started exploring alternative cooking methods beyond the bland boil and steam. Restaurants discovered they could fry the leaves, increasing oil absorption and creating a crunchier and nuttier flavor profile. Then they could add bacon, balsamic glaze, breadcrumbs, and parmesan cheese. Suddenly, it's not a humble vegetable. It's silky fat on sticky sugar on crunchy salt, layered to enhance richness, build desire, and make you say, "Damn, that's tasty."

The basic cooking principle is that sensory contrast makes food more exciting to eat. The more dynamic contrast—crispy paired with creamy, salty balanced with sweet—the more engaged our senses, and this stimulation makes it harder to stop eating.

This layering technique appears everywhere, such as in the crispy-creamy contrast of loaded cheese nachos, the soft-crunchy interplay of an Oreo cookie, or the crackling-silky combination of crème brûlée. These aren't random combinations. They are masterpieces of manipulating mouthfeel to make food more enjoyable.

Great chefs understand the value of strategically pairing salt, fat, acid, and heat. They recognize that monotony creates bland, uninspiring meals. But when a chef balances sweet and savory elements in a homemade meal, they work with whole ingredients whose flavors and textures naturally evolve during cooking. By contrast, when a food scientist engineers products in a corporate lab, they have one goal in mind: create the biggest craving possible.[10]

Food engineers use isolated compounds designed to trigger taste receptors with unnatural intensity. This is the difference between palatable food, such as Brussels sprouts you cook at home and top with nuts and honey, and hyperpalatable food, like Birds Eye Frozen Brussels Sprouts and Bacon Bake. The home-cooked version has three ingredients. The Birds Eye Brussels has thirty-three. One tastes good and is loaded with nutrients, the other tastes *too good*, turning what should be a normal eating experience into an overstimulated feedback loop. Hence the term hyperpalatable.

CALORIC DENSITY:
MORE ENERGY PACKED INTO EVERY BITE

Next time you're standing in your kitchen, try this experiment: Place a small bag of potato chips on the counter. Next to it, pile the four whole potatoes it took to make those chips. Now, imagine eating each pile in one sitting.

The chips? Gone in minutes, barely registering in your stomach, leaving you scanning the pantry for more. The whole potatoes? You'd be full halfway through the second one.

Same ingredient. Wildly different outcome.

While our ancestors worked to get more calories into their limited food supply, today's food concentrates enormous energy into tiny packages. They have high *caloric density*. A single fast-food meal can easily contain 1,500 calories—nearly a full day's energy requirements for many adults. The tablespoon of oil in your salad dressing contains 120 calories, while the dozens of olives required to produce it would fill you up long before delivering the equivalent amount of energy.

Understanding caloric density isn't about counting calories or doing complicated math. It's about recognizing when your body's ancient portion-control meter is being deliberately short circuited, and reclaiming your ability to feel genuinely satisfied with appropriate amounts of food.

THE DOPAMINE TRAP:
WHY PLEASURE HIJACKS OUR APPETITE

Dopamine isn't just about pleasure; it's about motivation. This neurotransmitter "wires" us to seek out and repeat experiences that feel good, reinforcing behaviors essential for survival. The issue is that in today's food environment, dopamine doesn't just nudge us toward sources of nourishment; it locks us into craving loops that are hard to escape.

In *The Compass of Pleasure*, David J. Linden, Ph.D., a professor of neuroscience at Johns Hopkins University, explains how pleasurable experiences set in motion a series of three processes that allow us to find repeatable satisfaction.[11]

Step 1. Pleasure hits you. You bite into something delicious— chocolate, pizza, ice cream—and a warm wave of satisfaction washes over you.

Step 2. Your nervous system stamps it. Your brain takes note of the taste, texture, and environment and associates them with happy thoughts and feelings, creating a pleasurable memory.

Step 3. Dopamine reinforces it. The next time you see, smell, or imagine that same food, dopamine is generated, urging you to seek it out again. The more dopamine is released, the more pleasant the memory, and the more effort you will expend to pursue this experience again.

This is why familiar foods trigger instant desire. Ever driven past a fast-food sign and suddenly "needed" fries? What about opening a bag of chips "for a few" and finishing the whole thing? That's dopamine at work, training your brain to crave foods before you even take a bite.

There's another powerful player involved in food rewards: endogenous opioids. These are natural, morphine-like chemicals your brain produces internally (*endogenous* simply means "from within") that create sensations of comfort, euphoria, and even mild pain relief. They're part of the same system activated by drugs like heroin, but in this case, they're produced by your body in response to food. This opioid response is especially strong for calorie-dense, highly palatable foods—the epitome of Food 2.0—and it helps explain why we often keep eating even when we're not hungry.[12]

When my son was scanning for samples at Costco on our last trip, these pleasurable neurochemicals were already at work in his nervous system. He was motivated to search for food because dopamine compelled him. Because he's had a stimulating eating experience previously, he was on a strong dopamine "roller-coaster ride" to recreate that rewarding experience.

Unfortunately, the larger the dopamine spike, the bigger the dip afterward. When you consume something extremely gratifying, your dopamine doesn't just rise and then return to normal; *it crashes, dropping way below baseline.*

What happens when your brain registers low dopamine? You start to feel a little glum, irritable, or restless. It's a nasty trick of our neurobiology. A moment ago, eating made you feel great. Now, you feel crummy. What gives?

The bigger problem is that these significant dopamine hits come with almost no effort. Nowadays, eating can be a mindless, hand-to-mouth motion, such as consuming a bag of chips, a candy bar, or a burger picked up at a drive-through window. As neuroscientist Andrew Huberman, Ph.D., says, having too much dopamine without exerting effort to obtain it is detrimental.[13] There's no chase, no waiting, or no energy expenditure. The exertion is gone but the rapture remains. The natural balance between effort and reward, a fundamental aspect of survival for millennia, has been completely thrown off.

"I WANT IT NOW": THE LOSS OF WAITING

From an evolutionary perspective, our inbuilt motivation-reward system made perfect sense. The combination of physical hunger and the dopamine-driven anticipation of reward pushed our ancestors to exert themselves to obtain food. Whether tracking an animal for miles, climbing a tree for fruit, or digging for tubers, there was always a gap between the desire to eat and the ability to satisfy that desire—effort preceded reward.

That gap is now gone.

Today, because our hunger and cravings can be instantly silenced, we undergo no struggle and burn no energy to acquire food. We just reach, unwrap, and chew.

Consider this from the perspective of your Inner Eaters, who are still operating on this ancient survival logic. Your Survival Eater evolved to maximize energy intake with minimal effort, a crucial survival strategy when food was scarce and required our ancestors to go hunting or foraging. But today, we're accumulating energy in quantities that are detrimental to our health. Calorie-dense Food 2.0 is more a liability than a lifesaver.

Meanwhile, your Pleasure Eater gets stuck on a hedonic treadmill. Eating hyperpalatable foods repeatedly stimulates the same reward pathways, which increases your threshold for enjoyment. Over time, pleasure becomes harder to elicit. Your taste buds lose their sensitivity to more subtle flavors. Your brain anticipates an explosion and feels let down when there's only a tiny pop. This is a frustrating scenario where the more you crave, the more you need to eat to experience that same high, and the less satisfying each bite becomes.

And when food requires zero effort to obtain, the cycle becomes even harder to break. Just like a smoker who reflexively reaches for a cigarette, your Pleasure Eater keeps reaching for the next bite—not out of hunger, but out of a fear, a sadness, or an anxiety you can't quite name. You can now soothe any unpleasant emotion with a reliable hit of mouth pleasure.

Your insatiable sweet tooth could just be your Pleasure Eater responding to a supermarket stocked with too-easy-to-get dopamine. Your endless hunger may be your Survival Eater detecting that something vital is missing from all this ultra-processed snack food—plenty of macronutrients, but not enough micronutrients to keep your cells happy.

When you see these external forces pulling apart your Inner Eaters, it gives you some space and grace. You're not helplessly broken. The system around you has irrevocably changed. Your Inner Eaters are reacting to this abnormal environment, asking to return to something familiar, but there is no going back. The challenge lies in how you lead them moving forward.

In Part Two of the book, you'll learn how to separate yourself from the reactions of your Inner Eaters. This will allow you to make new choices that better serve your conscious leadership and current reality. For now, practice noticing and naming your Inner Eaters as they show up. The first part of any transformation is building your awareness. Even if your Inner Eaters are hooked on Food 2.0, try not to pathologize them, they're doing the best they know how to keep you alive and safe. The more you understand the hijacks of Food 2.0, the easier it will be to manage your Eaters and bring them back to balance.

Hijack 2. Make It Effortless

I was walking through Cologne, Germany, with my wife when we passed a candy shop overflowing with jars of brightly colored gummy candies. My wife loves gummy bears, so we ducked inside, and she grabbed a small bag of the originals—Haribo® Goldbears®, made right there in Germany.

As she popped one in her mouth, she paused momentarily and said, "These are chewier than I remember." She wasn't imagining it. Haribo, the German confectioner who invented the gummy bear, specifically altered the texture for the American market. Their U.S. version is much softer and less chewy because, as one journalist put it in *The Atlantic*, "Americans don't really like to chew."[14]

And it's not just gummy bears. Across the board, the American food processing industry has shifted toward manufacturing softer,

45

more easily consumed foods. Food labels proclaiming "Now softer texture" appear on everything from protein bars to bread to beef jerky. This shift towards softness isn't just about texture preference; it has dramatic consequences for satiety, digestion, and the speed of eating.

PRECHEWED FOR YOUR CONVENIENCE

Chewing is the first step in digestion, and it was unavoidable for most of human history. Whole foods—fruits, vegetables, meats, and grains—required significant effort to break down. Chewing slowed the eating pace, giving the body time to recognize satiety signals and regulate intake. Our instincts tell us that we must keep chewing to get enough calories to keep our bodies alive.

But Food 2.0 engineers have taken chewing out of the eating equation.

Soft, ultraprocessed foods—from white bread to tenderized meats to one-minute rice—are designed to glide down with minimal effort. Whether instant oatmeal, protein shakes, or premashed, pulverized snacks, much of our food is essentially prechewed. This speeds up consumption and makes calories more concentrated and easier to absorb. The result? We eat faster and consume more before feeling full.[15]

In a groundbreaking study, when people ate ultraprocessed foods for two weeks, they consumed 500 more calories per day than when eating whole foods, without even realizing it.[16] The reason? As researchers concluded: "The softer food that was easier to chew and swallow led to increased eating rate and delayed satiety signaling, resulting in greater overall intake."[17]

VANISHING CALORIC DENSITY

"Some days I would get through my meal in a few minutes without really noticing I was eating. It wasn't satisfying."[18]

These are the reflections from a participant in the aforementioned ultraprocessed food study. He's pointing to an experience to which many of us can relate: eating without registering that we have eaten.

Food scientist Steven A. Witherly, Ph.D., has a name for this phenomenon: *vanishing caloric density*. According to Witherly, foods that "dissolve so quickly in your mouth so that your brain doesn't fully register the calories" encourage overconsumption.[19]

Here's how it works:

- The food melts instantly, so your mouth barely works (again, no chewing).

- Stretch receptors in your stomach never get activated, so your brain thinks you haven't eaten.

- Your microbiome becomes undernourished, so satiety signals get diminished or delayed.

- You keep eating because oral stimulation feels good, and your body has underestimated the calories you've consumed.

Without thinking, more than once I've eaten an entire bag of Bamba, my son's favorite peanut butter-flavored air-puffed snack. Each bite required no effort. Little chewing. Gone in a second. It was as if the whole bag just . . . vanished. Maybe you've had similar experiences with popcorn, ice cream, cheese puffs, or chocolate. All of these foods share a common characteristic of oral stimulation without stomach satiation.

Why is this an issue? Because eating is supposed to be a process, not just a transient experience of taste. When we strip away food's natural bulk and volume, the feedback loops between our guts and brains get disrupted. This is exactly why GLP-1 agonists, like Ozempic®, Wegovy®, and Mounjaro®, have surged in popularity. They trigger key satiety mechanisms that are otherwise lost due to the prechewed convenience and vanishing caloric density of Food 2.0.

THE RISE OF OZEMPIC AND OTHER GLP-1 AGONISTS

Drugs like Ozempic work by increasing GLP-1 (glucagon-like peptide-1), a hormone naturally produced in the gut that plays a crucial role in:

- Delaying gastric emptying. Slowing down digestion so food stays in the stomach longer, which dampens appetite and increases our feelings of fullness.

- Reducing appetite. Sending satiety signals to the brain alters hunger hormones and makes us feel satisfied with less food.

- Regulating blood sugar. Stimulating insulin production prevents us from having sugar spikes and crashes that drive ravenous eating.

Our gut-brain satiety system is designed by nature for a world of whole, fiber-rich foods that come from the earth and require lots of chewing (think tubers covered in dirt and seeds in thick shells). Food 2.0 broke this system. So we did exactly what modern society is good at: We designed a pharmaceutical solution to a humanmade problem.

There are many benefits to these drugs, and I expect their usage to soar over the coming years. People on GLP-1 agonists eat less because they feel full faster. They experience less hunger and less "food noise." Many report that for the first time in their lives, they feel free from obsessive food thoughts.[20]

For many struggling with their body weight or obesity, escaping the exhausting cycle of craving, resisting, and giving in can be a game changer. Clinical trials show that patients on GLP-1 agonists lose 10–15 percent of their body weight because they eat less without feeling deprived. In many ways, these drugs are brilliant tools. They give people the ability to experience satiety in a food environment that works against it.

These drugs do their job well, no question. But here's the biggest concern with over relying on a drug to manage your eating. These pharmaceuticals dampen the desire to eat but don't address our broken, unsustainable, chemically altered food system. If a user stops taking the drugs, hunger returns, and cravings creep back in. Then what? Food 2.0 is still everywhere, engineered for bliss points, hyperpalatability, and effortless overconsumption. The root cause of all these eating-related issues remains as strong as ever.

Without developing self-awareness about your Inner Eaters, you will miss the opportunity to create a sustainable, conscious relationship with food that works even when the medication you been taking (or are considering taking) isn't there anymore. Sure, you may lose weight by taking a GLP-1, but what about all the emotional baggage? What happens to years of body dissatisfaction, self-criticism, or preoccupation with food when your hunger returns?

A medication may dampen the voices of your Inner Eaters, but they're still there. Your Pleasure Eater's desire for comfort doesn't disappear; it becomes chemically subdued. Your Social Eater's need for connection through shared meals isn't addressed if you're too full to eat. Your Strategic Eater may celebrate weight loss without developing the skills to maintain it in the long term.

This is where Eating 2.0 provides something Ozempic cannot: It doesn't just mute hunger; it helps you understand it. When you undertake the real inner work of upgrading your eating habits, you become aware of how you habitually use food for pleasure, comfort, or reward. As the conscious leader of your own appetite, you get to decide how to integrate these patterns healthfully into your life.

GLP medications are not antagonistic to Eating 2.0. If your hunger is off the charts, a pharmaceutical might help regulate your voracious appetite, allowing you to start cultivating deeper wisdom about your eating. In this sense, GLP-1 agonists can create a valuable window of opportunity: a biochemical pause to do the real work of understanding who you are as an eater. The approach I'm recommending in this book isn't about forsaking technological tools or pursuing some path of purity; it's about helping you create sustainable transformation. For some individuals, that might require external supports like GLP-1s.

For those using or considering these medications, the question isn't whether you "should" (or "should not") take them—that's between you and your healthcare provider. The question is, will you use one of these new tools as a quick fix or as part of a more comprehensive approach to transform who you are as an eater?

Hijack 3. Make It Endless

The waiter set down the plate: a giant piece of white meat chicken flattened into a disk, coated with breadcrumbs, slathered with marinara and melted mozzarella, all atop angel hair pasta in an Alfredo-like cream sauce. My friend from Japan stared at it wide-eyed. It was his first time at the Cheesecake Factory, and the chicken parmesan in front of him looked like it could feed a family of four. "Wow, so much food," he said.

I just smiled and said, "Welcome to America."

Over the past fifty years, portion sizes have steadily crept upward, reshaping not only the plates in front of us but our very perception of what a meal should be—endless. Studies show that people tend to eat what's put in front of them, whether it's a sensible portion or a feast fit for a linebacker.[21] And the more we're exposed to oversized portions, the more they seem right, even expected.

This phenomenon, known as *portion distortion*, is one of the silent forces that hijack your Inner Eaters. It whispers to your Survival Eater, convincing it that today's standard meal is a reasonable amount of food. It entices your Pleasure Eater, presenting larger portions as a doorway to happiness. It reassures your Social Eater that piling the plate high is simply what people around here do. Your Strategic Eater? It gets blindsided when it realizes its "healthy" restaurant salad is 1,200 calories.

HOW WE GOT HERE

Portion sizes weren't always this way. In the 1970s, a standard fast-food soda was seven ounces. Today, the smallest size on many menus is sixteen ounces, with options going as high as sixty ounces—nearly a half-gallon of liquid sugar. In 1980, a standard bagel was about three inches in diameter; today, it's more than twice that size. The same goes for muffins, plates of pasta, and even steaks, which have ballooned in size at restaurants nationwide. A study from the *American Journal of Public Health* found that restaurant portions today are two to five times larger than in the 1950s.[22] The bigger issue is that these larger portions have recalibrated what Americans consider "normal."[23]

WHAT GOVERNS HOW MUCH WE EAT?

Think about the last time you ate at a restaurant. Did you finish everything on your plate? Did you feel full before the last bite (but kept eating anyway)? Did you pass the point of "no return," eating what's left rather than throwing it away or saving it for later?

The Clean Plate Club is a deeply ingrained cultural script that tells us to finish everything on our plates. Given that we evolved from hundreds of thousands of years of food scarcity, this "club" made a lot of sense. If you were raised in a family where leaving uneaten food on your plate was unacceptable, you probably have a membership card floating around somewhere.

There's something to be said about only taking as much food on your plate as you plan to eat. Practically nobody enjoys wasting food. However, believing that you must finish all the food on your plate can create many problems. Even if you don't consciously adhere to this rule, it seems that most people tend to eat the majority of the food they serve themselves, regardless of portion size.[24]

This tendency to eat to completion means that when portions grow, so does consumption, whether or not your body needs that much food. Psychologists attribute this behavior to a phenomenon known as *unit bias*. *Unit bias* refers to how we perceive a single unit of food, whether a sandwich, a bottled drink, or a prepackaged snack, as the appropriate amount to consume in one sitting. We like integers. We like completeness. This means that if a cookie is twice as large as a typical serving, most people will still eat the whole thing rather than stopping at half.[25]

Don't take my word for it. Test this in your own experience. When was the last time you ate one-fifth of a slice of pizza or four-fifths of a bagel?

CULTURAL COMPARISONS:
THE SUPERSIZED AMERICAN MEAL

Portion inflation is not universal. As my college friend from Japan demonstrated, what is considered normal in Japan differed significantly from the portion sizes at an American restaurant. In many countries, a "normal" meal is a fraction of what's served in the United States—modestly portioned proteins instead of twenty-ounce steaks, a small serving of cheese instead of giant cheese-pulls, one piece of bread rather than a sub sandwich on a whole loaf.[26]

I remember traveling to Thailand with my brother, where every meal we ordered took a long time to prepare. We joked that we had "overwhelmed the kitchen," not because we were demanding customers, but because we each ordered two, three, sometimes four dishes at a time. Accustomed to American portion sizes, we assumed we'd need more food to feel satisfied. When our plates arrived, the contrast was clear (and a little comical). What we considered a typical meal was far more significant than what Thai locals typically eat.

This experience highlighted an important truth: Portion sizes aren't just about hunger but about expectations. We don't just eat to satiety; we eat to match our internal sense of what "enough" feels like. If we anticipate that a dish, restaurant, or cuisine won't leave us feeling full, we preemptively order (and consume) more to compensate. Over time, this expectation reshapes our eating habits, stretching our definition of a proper meal and fueling the cycle of overconsumption.

THE CONFUSION OF NUTRITION LABELS

If portion inflation weren't enough, the way we measure food is equally deceptive. Until recently, many packaged foods listed "one serving" as an arbitrary fraction of the container—a trick that made calorie counts seem lower than they were. For example, a pint of ice cream was often labeled as four servings, even though few people would stop at a quarter of the container.

Recognizing this issue, the FDA updated nutrition labels in 2016 to reflect more realistic portion sizes. The new labels make it clear that a single bottle of soda or bag of chips is often not just one serving, helping consumers see the actual caloric impact.[27] Yet, even with these changes, old habits die hard. If we're accustomed to eating the whole package, knowing it contains multiple servings doesn't necessarily stop us from doing so.

THE "IMMORTALITY" OF MODERN FOOD

While portion sizes tell part of the story, the true "endlessness" of Food 2.0 goes far deeper. Consider this startling reality: Virtually nothing in a modern convenience store would spoil if left for months or years. This defiance of natural decomposition is no accident—it's engineering.

Unprocessed foods have natural life cycles. Milk sours, bread grows mold, fruits rot, and meat putrefies. These are natural signals that food shouldn't be consumed, a biological warning system that protected our ancestors.

Food 2.0, by contrast, exists in a strange biological limbo. Through the use of preservatives, stabilizers, and industrial processing techniques, these products resist the very forces of nature that would normally break them down. A typical packaged snack might contain calcium propionate to prevent mold, sodium benzoate to inhibit bacterial growth, BHA or BHT to prevent fats from going rancid, and sodium nitrite to maintain color. These chemical sentinels stand guard, ensuring packaged foods remain "good" long past their natural expiration date.

There is an obvious upside to all this unnatural shelf stability: more food options to choose from. However, in an environment where abundance never diminishes, it's easy to lose our bearings. Unlike ripening fruit that demands immediate attention, packaged foods can sit indefinitely—cookies in your pantry, frozen meals in your freezer, energy bars in desk drawers all remain "fresh" for months. Food 2.0 isn't bound by seasons, geography, or time, and this means there are few natural guardrails limiting how much you eat.

FRAGMENTED INTO ENDLESS VARIETY

Beyond supersizing and immortalizing food, the industry has mastered another dimension of endlessness: fragmenting foods into seemingly infinite variations. Where once there were simply potato chips, now entire aisles are dedicated to dozens of flavors, textures, shapes, and formulations of the same basic product.

This endless proliferation serves a dual purpose. First, it creates the illusion of novelty without nutritional improvement. Your Inner Eaters, particularly your Pleasure Eater, are drawn to the promise of new experiences—salt and vinegar today, jalapeño tomorrow, and honey barbecue the day after. Each variation feels like a distinct choice rather than repetitive consumption of the same ultraprocessed product.

Second, it ensures that no matter how specific your preferences, there's a product engineered exactly for you. Gluten sensitive but craving cookies? There's a version for that. Want protein-enhanced ice cream? It exists. Looking for sugar-free, low-carb crackers that taste like pizza? Someone makes those, too. The message is clear: Food 2.0 has no natural limitations; only endless options tailored precisely to your desires.

THE COST OF ENDLESSNESS

This engineered endlessness comes with profound costs to our physiological and psychological well-being. Our digestive systems have evolved to process foods that decompose—foods containing enzymes, fiber structures, and microorganisms that work in conjunction with our gut bacteria to support proper digestion and immune function. Consuming predominantly shelf-stable, ultraprocessed foods deprives our microbiome of the diverse inputs it needs to maintain balance.

The psychological cost is equally significant. When food never spoils, never runs out, and comes in endless varieties, our Inner Eaters become overwhelmed and stressed. This creates what psychologist Barry Schwartz calls the *paradox of choice*. Despite being surrounded by more food options than ever in human history, many of us experience a persistent sense that we might miss out on something better, newer, or more satisfying just around the corner.[28] This results in both anxiety—*Did I choose the best option?* —and regret—*I should have ordered the other dish*. Food advertisements exacerbate this "food FOMO," keeping us in a constant state of mild dissatisfaction and craving something better. Sadly, this is precisely where the food industry wants us— unhappy and hungry for more.

Understanding the engineered endlessness of Food 2.0 is crucial to reclaiming a healthier relationship with eating. By recognizing how unnatural perpetual abundance is, we can estab- lish our own boundaries and rhythms that honor our body's actual needs rather than the industry's need for endless consumption.

Food 2.0 vs. Our Inner Eaters

Walk into a modern grocery store, airport terminal, or gas station, and your Inner Eaters get bombarded. Your Pleasure Eater perks up at the sight of chocolate-dipped protein bars. Your Survival Eater gets triggered by the smell of bacon wafting through the air. Your Strategic Eater scans nutrition labels, hoping to assert control, but becomes paralyzed in analysis. Your Inner Eaters are caught between two worlds: looking for something they recognize and finding only Food 2.0.

Consider this: In 1700, England's average sugar intake was four pounds per year—about one teaspoon daily. Today? One hundred and fifty pounds per year. That's three-quarters of a cup of sugar per person daily, over 500 calories.[29]

In 2010, Americans had access to roughly 4,000 calories per day—double what most people need.[30] That's 1.46 million calories per year, just for you!

Living in a world of surplus calories changes how we operate. We snack more often. We eat larger portions. We choose indulgence more freely. The interesting part is that we don't even notice it happening because the environment makes it feel normal.

Our bodies have a perfect way to handle surplus calories: Convert them into fat. And they do this dutifully, assuming famine is coming, just as it was for most of human evolution.

This is why obesity is such a huge issue. One study predicts that 256 million people in the United States will be overweight or obese by 2050.[31] That's one in three adolescents and two out of every three adults. The disease burden and economic costs will be devastating. Yet, despite the growing problem, we keep eating—not out of necessity, but because Food 2.0 makes it easy, expected, and ingrained in the modern way of life.

This isn't about assigning blame or shame to individuals. The system is designed to make extra calories as delicious as possible. There's so much delicious food available, that if a food is located in your home, founder of Precision Nutrition, John Berardi, Ph.D., quips, "Either you, someone you love, or someone you marginally tolerate will eventually eat it."[32]

Understanding how this system works—from the fifty-ingredient frozen dinner to the psychological manipulation that gets it into your cart—is the first step toward making different choices. The next step is understanding how this environment of perpetual stimulation, effortless access, and endless availability impacts your Inner Eaters.

YOUR SURVIVAL EATER: NO BRAKES, NO BOUNDARIES

Your Survival Eater evolved to ensure your body has adequate nutrition, always seeking maximum return on effort. But Food 2.0 requires virtually no effort. It's precut, precooked, blended, stripped of fiber, mechanically processed, and infinitely shelf stable. It arrives ready to eat and can wait patiently for weeks, months, or even years until you're ready to consume it. This unprecedented combination of convenience and preservation obliterates the natural constraints that once regulated consumption.

The point isn't to demonize modern food technology. Pre-chopped vegetables, preportioned proteins, and ready-to-go meal kits offer genuine benefits in our overscheduled world. I rely on these conveniences to feed myself and my family. However, without natural boundaries of spoilage or effort, we must accept that our Survival Eaters may get caught in a feast that never ends. Over time, they may become accustomed to nothing less.

YOUR PLEASURE EATER:
TRAPPED IN A CYCLE OF CRAVING

Engineered bliss points flood your Pleasure Eater with artificial reward, creating dopamine cycles that promise satisfaction but never deliver. Each bite triggers cravings for the next, keeping you perpetually unsatisfied.

Remember that snack that dissolves instantly in your mouth? That endless supermarket shelf: dozens of chip flavors, cereal varieties, and beverage options? All this sensory bombardment intrigues your Pleasure Eater, creating an eating experience so far beyond natural parameters that your Pleasure Eater can never find enough. The worst part is that the goalposts of "enough" keep shifting as your neurochemistry adapts to expect ever-greater stimulation.

YOUR STRATEGIC EATER:
FIGHTING AN UNWINNABLE WAR

Your Strategic Eater evolved for caloric abundance, but Food 2.0 uses clever marketing and nutritional sleight of hand to scramble its good intentions. Food companies fortify ultraprocessed products with protein and vitamins, creating "health halos" that fool your Strategic Eater into thinking engineered foods are nutritious choices.

A vitamin-fortified breakfast cereal is still a sugar delivery system. A protein-packed cookie is still a cookie. Energy bars marketed as "clean" are engineered to taste like dessert while containing stabilizers, texturizers, and sweeteners designed to trick you into believing you're eating something you're not. These "functional" foods lure your Strategic Eater with health promises while retaining opiate-triggering compounds that lead to overconsumption.

This creates an endless arms race where the food industry first profits from selling hyperpalatable products, then profits again by marketing supposedly healthier alternatives to fix the problems they created. What's worse, they fund research designed to obscure these connections, leaving consumers constantly chasing the next nutritional breakthrough that never quite delivers lasting health.

I'm not suggesting all food engineering is harmful. The problem isn't the technology itself but how it's deployed in the service of endless consumption rather than genuine nourishment. Your Strategic Eater can leverage food innovations intelligently, but only when operating from educated awareness rather than reacting to industry-driven narratives.

YOUR SOCIAL EATER: ISOLATED AND OVERWHELMED

While the physical properties of Food 2.0 directly impact your Pleasure, Survival, and Strategic Eaters, your Social Eater faces a different but equally profound challenge: the severing of food's traditional role in community and relationships.

The Social Eater evolved for a world where eating was communal, yet Food 2.0 offers endless individually packaged products designed for solo consumption. Eating alone while scrolling our phone screens has become the norm. Meanwhile, labels for styles of eating, such as "vegan" or "keto," have created new social identities that leave your Social Eater perplexed and wondering if you too should "join the club."

Looking Ahead:
Culturally Condoned Overeating

Understanding how Food 2.0 systematically hijacks your Inner Eaters is the first step toward reclaiming agency and power. You're not fighting fair odds. You're fighting a system engineered to exploit every survival instinct that once kept you alive.

But Food 2.0's biological manipulation is only half the battle. The other half is cultural. Eating has become a 24/7 experience mediated by screens, stress, and social pressure. Food has become performance art, and Instagramable meals have become status symbols.

That's where we'll go next. Let's see how the culture of Food 2.0 hijacks your Inner Eaters and makes healthy eating more challenging than ever.

TWO

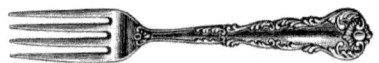

WHEN DINNER BROKE

THE THREE DISRUPTIONS THAT FOREVER CHANGED HOW YOU EAT

"There was a time, if you can believe it, when a respectable person could not have a little treat whenever she wanted. This time was, roughly, from the dawn of the republic to the middle of the 1980s."

ELLEN CUSHING

Hazel steps into her kitchen—though to call it a *kitchen* stretches the meaning of the word. It's no longer a place for cooking, just an area for assembling and reheating. She's running late, so breakfast is a croissant and coffee sipped between emails. By noon, she's deep in a work sprint, smartphone in one hand, scrolling through messages on its screen while absently crunching on some crackers she grabbed from the pantry.

Lunch? She hadn't planned anything. She rarely does. Maybe she'll heat up something later, maybe not. There are plenty of leftovers in the fridge and a freezer full of microwavable meals.

By late afternoon, Hazel realizes she's barely moved from her desk. A quick energy boost is needed. She reaches for a granola bar, then a handful of M&Ms. She's not even sure if she's hungry or just bored. When she's busy working, eating kinda just *happens*.

Dinnertime arrives, but it doesn't feel like a meal. It's a patchwork of bites—some cheese while she preps her son's dinner, some leftovers straight from the fridge, and then a few chips while watching a show. No plates, no ceremony, just food absorbed into the flow of the day.

Hazel pauses for a second, staring at the empty counter. She remembers Sunday dinners at her grandmother's house—the smell of slow-cooked stew, the clatter of plates, the feeling of being full and satisfied in a way that had nothing to do with calories. The moment passes. Now she feels empty and heads to the fridge for one more bite without thinking. She never really stops to eat anymore.

And she's not alone.

The New Normal:
Always Eating, Never Nourished

While the previous chapter explored how food companies deliberately hijack our biology. The transformation of our eating habits runs deeper than ultraprocessed ingredients or newfangled packaging. We're not just eating different foods; we're eating in a fundamentally different way.

Three fundamental cultural disruptions have reshaped our entire relationship with eating. These are:

- **Snack life**. We've shifted from mealtimes to always-on grazing.

- **Mindless eating.** We've gone from looking at our food to looking at our screens.

- **Status bites.** We've gone from food as nourishment to social broadcasting, virtue signaling, and plate politics.

Food manufacturers may have loaded the gun with ultra-processed, portable, hyperpalatable snacks, but these cultural forces pulled the trigger. The reframing of hunger, the collapse of mealtime rituals, and the normalization of multitasking have detached eating from time, place, and community.

No single company or marketing campaign created this reality. Yet together, modern food systems and lifestyles have engineered a world where eating is constant, yet connection is absent; appetite is everywhere, yet satisfaction is elusive. This is the cultural disruption of Food 2.0, and while it may feel convenient or normal, it carries profound consequences for your body, mind, and identity.

Disruption 1. Snack Life

Remember when dinner was dinner—a designated time when people gathered, shared food, and then finished eating until the next day? Today, that ritual has vanished.

In 2006, USDA researchers added a new category to their studies: *all-day eating.*[1] Their research showed that the old categories—*primary eating* (meals with full attention) and *secondary eating* (eating while doing something else like watching TV)—no longer captured reality. Mealtimes had blurred into a steady hum of grazing all day long.

We've become a nation of snackers. We pop protein bars during meetings, munch while waiting in line, and scroll with one hand while reaching for a bite with the other. What once would have seemed rude or indulgent now feels routine. Roughly one-quarter of Americans' calories now come from snacks.[2] Our modern food culture tells us: if you feel hungry, even for a moment, you should satisfy it. And thanks to Food 2.0, we can.

Before the twentieth century, eating away from home was rare and done only out of necessity. In fact, a hundred years ago, the need to eat away from home was *tolerated as an inconvenience.* Meals that were eaten out were social rituals—weddings, funerals, and celebrations. Even in these situations, attendees often brought food from their homes. Eating out was still essentially homemade.

Nowadays, no one has time to cook, or rather, our modern food system has created a world where cooking no longer feels necessary. Instead of cooking, people assemble meals from endless grab-and-go options prepared by invisible laborers in factories and backrooms. Eating patterns have become like our social media feeds: always pinging for our attention, heavily influenced by ads, and deceptively unsatisfying. As Hazel's day demonstrates, when all-day snacking becomes normal, your Inner Eaters rarely ever feel truly full or truly hungry.

The normalcy of anywhere-anytime eating is startling in its completeness. Ninety-three percent of Americans report snacking daily, with 70 percent of Millennials admitting to replacing at least one daily meal with snacks.[3] Americans now spend 54 percent of food budgets on meals prepared outside the home (an all-time high), almost double what people spent in 1970.[4]

Corporate culture has accelerated this shift away from square meals to all-day grazing. Office kitchens overflow with snacks. "Desktop dining" has become normal. You know what that's like: one hand on the keyboard, the other clutching a sandwich.[5] Taking a full lunch hour often feels indulgent, even lazy.

You might be thinking, *Why is this a problem? I like my snacks. I enjoy being productive during the day and have no issues forgoing bigger meals.*

I have no issue with snacking either, except for this: Our societal shift from structured eating to constant consumption shapes *what* and *how much* we eat. Snacks are, by definition, transitional items to curb hunger between meals. When we increase our snack intake (without subsequently decreasing our meal intake), we end up eating more calories with fewer nutrients. We now live in a perpetual buffet of snacks that keep hunger at bay but lower the overall quality of our diet. Moreover, they undermine our ability to sit with the mild discomfort of being hungry—turning a perfectly natural human experience into something to be vanquished.

THE RISE OF SNACKIFICATION

Why does grabbing a bag of chips feel much easier than sitting down for a real meal? There's actually a hidden economic force at play. In most states, that bag of chips isn't taxed, but if you order the same amount of food as a meal at a restaurant, you'll pay sales tax. Decades of food industry lobbying have deliberately shaped these tax policies to keep processed snack foods artificially cheap. Meanwhile, federal agricultural subsidies make the corn, soybeans, and wheat that form the backbone of snack foods artificially inexpensive.

The result is the rise of "snackification," where artificially cheap processed foods have crowded out nutritious meals from our daily eating patterns, and the food industry profits enormously from this shift. Every snack represents another purchase opportunity. Many foods that used to be eaten at mealtimes have been repackaged as snacks for convenience. For example, pizza has become bite-sized Bagel Bites® (Heinz), peanut butter sandwiches have become crustless, sealed Uncrustables® (Smucker's), and yogurt has been put in squeezable tubes for on-the-go eating (there are a few competing brands).

This explains something your Strategic Eater has probably noticed: companies have engineered a snack-dominated grocery ecosystem, with entire aisles devoted to on-the-go products. The food industry has spent millions ensuring that grabbing processed snacks remains the path of least resistance with the highest profit margins. When California tried to change this in 1991 by taxing snacks as luxuries, the food industry poured over $2 million into repealing the law. Within a year, it was gone.[6]

The result? When your Survival Eater is tired and looking for quick fuel, it's not choosing between equal options; it's choosing in a system designed to optimize impulse-driven purchases and nudge you toward the snack aisle. Food companies have successfully monetized our basic fear of starvation on an unprecedented scale.

HOW YOUR INNER EATERS LOSE THEIR GUARDRAILS

Since the snackification of America shows little sign of reversing, it's important to recognize the consequences on your Inner Eaters.

Your Survival Eater adapts to snackification. When food is always accessible, your Survival Eater loses tolerance for even mild hunger, reaching for snacks at the first hint of discomfort. The issue is that a move toward snacking often means a diet with more energy-dense foods, added sugars, refined starches, sodium, and unhealthy fats, as well as less protein, fiber, and micronutrients compared to full meals.

Your Pleasure Eater mistakes stimulation for satisfaction. Flavor is never far away, but true pleasure, the kind that comes from anticipation, ritual, and savoring, becomes harder to access. There's no beginning, buildup, or climax, just a blur of bites— paradoxically leading some to eat *more* by continuously chasing *full*-fillment.

Your Social Eater loses connection. Americans spend more time dining alone than at any point in history.[7] Without conversation to pace the meal or others to share with, eating often becomes lonely or rushed. When families no longer eat together at set times, individuals (especially children and teens) may constantly nibble on snack foods without ever having a balanced meal. Let's get real: In a Food 2.0 world, kids aren't reaching for broccoli or kale; they're reaching for whatever cartoon characters call "cool," or whatever their favorite athlete pretends to eat on TikTok.

Your Strategic Eater thrives on efficiency. *A sit-down meal? Wasteful. A few random bites between meetings? Optimal.* This line of thinking thrives in a culture that sees mealtimes as obstacles to more important tasks, diminishing the value of eating itself. A balanced meal (say, a plate with protein, vegetables, and whole grains) might be replaced by a series of snack items that, even if calorically similar, are nutritionally poor.

Some days, snacks on-the-go might be precisely what you need. At other times, a genuine meal, following social rhythms—even just a few mindful bites—might bring you more peace, health, and harmony than fragmented bites. The invitation is not to disband with snacks, but to make these choices consciously rather than defaulting to the food industry's stealth snackification or hustle culture's micro-fueling to support productivity.

Disruption 2. Mindless Eating

Think about your last meal: Did you notice when you felt full? Did you look at your food? Can you describe three sensory experiences from it?

If you're drawing a blank, you're not alone. Most of us eat on autopilot, missing the very experience our bodies are designed to savor. When meals dissolve into background activities, we become disconnected from the sensory experience of eating. Attention splits between screens, tasks, and the next thing to do, rather than the food itself.

Research confirms the cost: People who eat while distracted consume 10 percent more in one sitting and are 25 percent more likely to overeat later.[8] Satiety isn't just physical—it's psychological. Our brains need to register the eating experience to feel satisfied.

Eating can be one of the most visceral, sensory-rich experiences of being alive: Recall the warmth of fresh bread in your hands, the crisp snap of an apple, or the smoothness of dark chocolate melting on your tongue. However, instead of feeling the textures, tasting the layers of flavor, and noticing when we're satisfied, Food 2.0 is designed to be consumed in a fog of disconnection. Awareness only returns when we hit the bottom of the bag, the last spoonful, or the empty plate. It's like waking up from a dream. *Wait, did I just eat all of that?*

SCREENS AS OUR DINING COMPANIONS

The average American sees over 2,000 food ads per year—nearly six daily.[9] Fast-food commercials showcase melted cheese pulls and slow-motion sauce dunking, perfectly designed to stimulate brain reward circuits that make you want to eat. It's not just that more people are eating in front of screens, it's that those screens are selling you hunger, and within seconds, also giving you options to satisfy that hunger. Ever wonder why an ad for Uber Eats or DoorDash appears immediately after an ad for McDonald's or Coca-Cola? It's to stimulate desire.

The irony is almost too rich: We eat microwaved dinners while watching celebrity chefs prepare elaborate feasts. We scroll through perfect Instagram plates while eating from plastic containers. We consume food content as entertainment, but our own meals feel rushed and forgettable.

This is the paradox of eating in a Food 2.0 world: When we're glued to screens, we eat more but enjoy it less, creating what researchers call a *pleasure deficit.*[10]

Here's what happens: Even if you just had a big, tasty meal, when you fail to notice the pleasure because you were distracted, your brain still screams out in hunger. Your Pleasure Eater never met its needs, so it asks for more. But often, it's too late. The meal is over. The actual pleasure is gone. So what does your brain do? It reaches for another distracted bite, hoping this time will be different.

Your Social Eater gets confused, too: *Am I eating with these people on my screen* or *just salivating while Gordon Ramsay yells at someone else's risotto?* Your Strategic Eater tries to multitask but ends up doing neither activity well. Meanwhile, your Survival Eater sees all these food images and mistakes them for reality, revving up your appetite without actually paying attention to the food you have. No wonder you can eat an entire plate and still be thinking about food a minute later. Mindless consumption is like watching a movie while staring at your phone the whole time—you "saw" it, but you didn't experience it.

THE STRESS-SLEEP-HUNGER SPIRAL

It's 11 PM. You're finally done with work, sprawled on the couch with your laptop still on your chest. Your brain buzzes from the day's chaos, but your body feels drained. You know you should go to bed, but instead, you find yourself scrolling your phone while mindlessly reaching for whatever's in arm's reach—crackers, leftovers, that snack that's been sitting in your pantry for who knows how long.

Late-night snacking is a common complaint I hear again and again from the clients in my men's wellness coaching practice. While there are many reasons for this habit, two things in particular exacerbate it: chronic stress and sleep deprivation. When you feel overwhelmed, whether from work pressure, social media, or the constant stream of troubling news, your nervous system responds as if you are in physical danger. Then, dump all that stress into a nervous system that hasn't gotten enough sleep, and you create a biological cascade that fundamentally alters how you eat.

Because you're stressed, your body releases too much cortisol, which not only increases your appetite, but also specifically drives your cravings for high-calorie "comfort" foods.[11] If stress is persistent, over time, two additional effects may occur. Your gut microbiome shifts, and the "stop" signals that tell you you've had enough grow weaker. Your hormones become imbalanced: Ghrelin (the "hunger hormone") increases while leptin (the "fullness hormone") decreases. The result is more "gas" and fewer "brakes" on your appetite.[12]

But here's what makes late-night eating particularly problematic: It's not just about the extra calories; it's about timing.

Your body doesn't just track what you eat; it tracks when you eat. Every cell in your body operates on an internal clock, synchronized to the rhythm of light and darkness. Your metabolism, hormone production, and digestive capacity fluctuate predictably throughout the day, optimized for different functions at different times. These patterns are your *circadian rhythms.*

For hundreds of thousands of years, humans typically ate when the sun was up and fasted when it went down. This wasn't a lifestyle choice; it was a necessity. Without artificial light or refrigeration, nighttime meant danger and scarcity. Your ancestors couldn't DoorDash a midnight snack or raid the fridge at 2 AM. When darkness fell, the world became more dangerous, and it was time to shelter in place, stop eating, and allow the body to enter rest and repair mode.

Your digestive system still operates on this ancient schedule. During daylight hours, your body produces more digestive enzymes, your metabolism increases, and your insulin sensitivity peaks. As evening approaches, these systems naturally wind down, preparing for the overnight fast that allows your body to focus on cellular repair, memory consolidation, and restoration.

Eating late at night is like sending your body an unexpected package after business hours—it doesn't quite know what to do with it. That's why that bowl of pasta at noon and the same bowl at midnight affect your body differently. Research confirms this: Identical meals eaten at night versus earlier in the day are more likely to contribute to weight gain and metabolic dysfunction.[13]

This is why that 11 PM snack attack is as much a biology problem as a lifestyle problem. Tired bodies crave quick fuel, sleepy brains lose decision-making capacity, and your Inner Eaters get scrambled by mixed messages between what your biology expects (rest) and what your environment offers (endless food availability). Your Survival Eater is trying to solve an energy crisis, but what you actually need is sleep. Your Strategic Eater knows you should go to bed, but it's too exhausted to override your Survival Eater's demands.

Instead of beating yourself up for eating late at night, you can ask yourself: *What do my Inner Eaters actually need right now?* Often, it's not more food; it's earlier bedtimes, better stress management, or simply recognizing that 11 PM hunger might be burnout in disguise.

WHEN YOUR INNER EATERS GET SCRAMBLED

Think back to Hazel reaching for a granola bar and nuts as she stares at her computer screen. Despite her second coffee, she feels the familiar afternoon energy crash. Her Survival Eater makes what seems like a logical connection: *I'm exhausted. My body needs energy. I should eat something.* She doesn't realize that her Survival Eater isn't asking for calories; it's desperately signaling for something food can't provide—nervous system regulation and genuine rest.

This is a fundamental confusion: mistaking the body's call for recovery as a call for fuel. It keeps many people caught in a cycle of stress-eating that never addresses the root cause. As a result:

- Your **Survival Eater** will overcompensate when tired, reaching for quick, easy options as a substitute for deep restoration.

- Your **Pleasure Eater** will seek comfort in familiar flavors, usually a sweet fix, and will use mouth stimulation as a respite from exhaustion.

- Your **Social Eater** might look around only to find everyone else working, sleeping, or sitting on the couch, eating a snack with you.

- Your **Strategic Eater** will struggle to operate in a sleep-deprived state. It can try to track every macronutrient, but it can't override your body's internal clock. Even healthy food, eaten at the wrong time, hits differently.

The cruel irony is that the more exhausted you become, the less capable you will be of leading your Inner Eaters. The mental clarity needed to recognize them in action disappears. Instead of seeing them, *you become them*—raw impulses steering without awareness. So the pattern repeats: stress, exhaustion, mindless snacking, staying up too late, poor sleep, and waking up already depleted.

Next time you feel the urgent need to snack during a stressful afternoon or late at night, pause and ask: *Do my Inner Eaters need more calories or are they really tired and stressed?* They may be begging for another bite, but that is because they don't know how to ask for what they truly need: a deep breath and a moment of rest.

If your stress never relents, your Inner Eaters will continue to seek safety where they can find it, constantly chasing the next bite, hoping for a moment of relief. The key to breaking this cycle is not with more control but more compassion. These parts of you want you to feel safe, but the more stressed out you are, the less able you are to give them tender love and care. What they really need is proof that you're safe enough to slow down. But most of us don't even realize how wound up we are until the moment we finally stop and notice how hard it is to actually rest. Food 2.0 doesn't support that kind of deep recovery. It wants you wired, tired, and reaching for the next bite.

Disruption 3. Status Bites

Scrolling through Instagram, I paused on a photo of an açai bowl topped with artfully arranged fruit and edible flowers. The caption read: "Starting my day with CLEAN fuel! #wellness #eatclean #blessed."

I sighed, thinking about my breakfast earlier that day, a hastily grabbed protein bar. I knew I "should" be fasting until noon, making chia smoothies, or scrambling avocado eggs, but somehow this never happens. I could feel the familiar weight of food judgment settling in. *Who am I if I'm not living up to the ideals of health and wellness that I see all over social media? What if people knew I eat protein bars for breakfast?*

This is the final disruption of our modern food landscape: Eating has become performative. There's an ecosystem of judgment, status, and identity wrapped around every bite. These "status bites" are then photographed, filtered, hashtagged, and broadcast for everyone to see.

THE RISE OF DIET TRIBES

I have friends who swear by keto, others who are deep in the vegan movement, and colleagues who have gone full paleo after watching one too many Joe Rogan video clips. Each group speaks about their way of eating as if it were more than just a diet—it is a worldview, a badge of honor, and a secret handshake that signals belonging.

At dinner parties, announcing dietary restrictions has replaced small talk about the weather. "So what do you eat . . . or rather, what *don't* you eat?" has become the question of our age. Announcing your dietary identity—be it grain-free, dairy-free, seed oil-free, or gluten-free—isn't just about naming your preferences; it's a performance of your values, health consciousness, environmental concerns, and social status.

Your diet commitments signal everything: Are you disciplined (*low-carb, sugar-free, intermittent fasting*)? Are you ethical (*vegan, organic, locally sourced*)? Are you primal (*grass-fed meat, raw dairy, no seed oils*)? Every food choice is a public statement.

It's not just what you eat; it's what you wear. In many social circles, especially among men, wearing a brewery's logo on your tee-shirt or cap is as common as sporting a band logo or a hometown sports team's jersey. I've got my fair share of brewery shirts, which I collected on road trips, like souvenirs from famous landmarks. These garments are identity markers.

A hazy IPA shirt says, "I know my hops and I support local." A whiskey distillery hat nods to rugged individualism and old-school masculinity. Even your takeout bag carries semiotic weight: Do you align more with the eco-conscious aesthetic of Sweetgreen salads or the meat-loving authenticity of smokehouse BBQ? To eat in the twenty-first century is to constantly broadcast who you are, what you value, and which tribe you belong to.

WHEN FOOD BECOMES MORALITY

When eating becomes a performance of who you are (or who you aspire to be), eating stops being simple. That cookie isn't just a snack; it's evidence of moral superiority or moral failing. It depends on whether you purchased it at the local farmers' market, made by hand with organic ingredients, or from the 50 percent off aisle at Kroger. One carries the image of purity; the other carries the weight of mass-produced inferiority. Even if the cookies are nutritionally identical, the simple pleasure of nourishment gets buried under layers of judgment, comparison, and anxiety.

This moralization of food has real consequences. Firstly, studies show labeling foods "forbidden" triggers the what-the-hell effect: *What the hell, I've already blown it. Might as well finish the bag.* Minor indulgences can lead to a complete abandonment of one's intentions.[14] You have one bite of something you've decided is "off limits," feel like you've broken the rules, and then spiral. This reaction is a predictable psychological loop triggered by restriction. It is your Strategic Eater collapsing under impossible standards and your Survival Eater stepping in to take the slack. The result is ending your meal with remorse, turning a "bad food day" into feelings of unworthiness.

Secondly, while traditional food ethics were rooted in collective values—cleanliness, honor, reverence—modern food morality often revolves around *individual* purity and status. Religious dietary laws, such as the kosher and halal rules, connect food to sacred rituals, community belonging, and spiritual alignment. In many eastern traditions, vegetarianism emerged not from a trend but from deeply held beliefs about nonviolence and compassion toward animals.

What's new isn't the idea that food choices have moral implications; it's the way these considerations have been coopted by marketing, stripped of their cultural contexts, and transformed into personal virtue signaling. The notion of "clean" eating is less a reflection of cultural wisdom and more a performance of self-discipline. Organic, gluten-free, glyphosate-free, and non-GMO are branding reframed as lifestyle credentials. "No seed oils" has become shorthand for signaling that you're "in the know" and a host of other ideas about "health."[15]

In a world where many feel disconnected from shared moral frameworks, food has become one of the few remaining terrains where people seek to locate meaning, identity, and goodness. Like political tribalism or religious affiliation, dietary identity offers a sense of righteousness. But without a coherent narrative of shared purpose or collective care, these food identities often devolve into forms of performative isolation—attempts to patch a deeper moral hunger with labels and lifestyle codes.[16]

The Food 2.0 culture amplifies eating as a performance of virtue, value, and social standing. (Hence: status bites.) The message is clear: "Buy this product, become this person," "Eat this way, and join a special group of people who have 'figured it out.'" Celebrity endorsements are a prime example. Post pictures of your meals online, receive affirmation that you're "eating the *right* way." The inquiry is whether upholding a socially desirable identity through food makes eating more or less enjoyable. I don't have the answer, but I do know it's hard to enjoy your lunch when you're busy angling for the best photo of it.

THE PRIVILEGE PARADOX

If you've ever felt like you're "doing healthy eating wrong," here's something that might help: The images of wellness you see online aren't just unrealistic, they're often suspiciously White, expensive, and completely inaccessible.[17]

That $14 turmeric latte? That's an ancient Indian healing drink, repackaged and marked up 500 percent. Bone broth, fermented vegetables, roasted seaweed, and sprouted grains have nourished families for generations, long before they became Instagram-worthy "superfoods." Foods once dismissed as "ethnic," "smelly," or "weird" are now repackaged as trendy. What was once mocked becomes marketable.

This matters for your Inner Eaters because it explains why eating healthy can feel so foreign, or expensive. Your Inner Eaters evolved in food cultures that were coherent, relational, and passed down from one nonna, abuela, or bubbe at a time—foods chosen not for macros but for memory, flavor, healing, and survival. Your Social Eater might feel pressure to eat like a wellness influencer, but the foods that sustained your grandparents probably contain more wisdom than any trendy green powder.

This isn't about bashing superfoods or blaming people for buying probiotic snacks from Instagram. It's about asking ourselves, "Who gets credit? Who gets paid? And who gets erased?" Something gets lost when ancient foods are stripped of context and sold back to us as trendy wellness breakthroughs. The line between cultural appropriation and cultural appreciation gets blurred when ancient "better for you" ingredients are marketed with drool-worthy images that attract your attention and evoke your desire.

And then there's the matter of access. The goal of eating "clean" assumes you have the time to prepare twelve-ingredient chia puddings, can buy fresh produce, or use a kitchen stocked with the appropriate tools or organic vegetables. Not everyone has those things. When food morality ignores our realities, it turns systemic barriers—like food deserts, poverty, shift work, and multigenerational caregiving—into personal failures. If the only version of "healthy" you ever see requires access to a Whole Foods, fancy powders, and protein shakes, you're not seeing the whole picture.

What is the result of this "Whitewashed" wellness world? Many people feel judged or ashamed, not because they're eating poorly, but because they don't *look* like the curated version of health they see online. This is where your Strategic Eater absorbs toxic messaging, your Pleasure Eater gets confused between genuine desire and mimetic desire—desiring what others have—and your Social Eater starts asking, *Do I even belong at the table?*

HOW PERFORMATIVE EATING HIJACKS YOUR INNER EATERS

Food 2.0 is designed to keep you overthinking your food choices, worrying if you're "doing it right," and performing for others, all at the same time. While food has always been entangled with status, religion, and identity, what's different today is how hyper-individualism and social media shape eating. Your Inner Eaters get caught in this performance, creating internal conflict about what, when, and how you should eat. As a result:

- Your **Survival Eater** may push you toward "safe" foods it grew up eating or foods that won't trigger shame or judgment. Deep down, it doesn't understand all the performative hubbub. *Why is quinoa considered better than rice? If it's safe to eat, let's eat!*

- Your **Pleasure Eater** gets confused by conflicting messages. *Should I enjoy that slice of cake or feel guilty about it? Is eating that burger making me happy or killing the planet?* The constant moral evaluation can dampen your ability to experience genuine satisfaction, leaving you either rigidly restricted or rebelliously indulgent.

- Your **Social Eater** faces a minefield at every gathering. *Will my dietary choices mark me as difficult, righteous, or simply different?* The fear of judgment—both giving and receiving it—transforms communal eating into a site of anxiety.

- Your **Strategic Eater** becomes overzealous, constantly calculating whether each bite aligns with your chosen dietary identity. It turns eating into a complex algorithm of virtue points, social media likes, and approval seeking rather than health or satisfaction.

The Cost of Living in Food 2.0

Step back and consider what we've lost in this transformation. The three disruptions of Food 2.0—snack life, mindless eating, and status bites—have fundamentally altered our relationship with eating itself, leaving many people stuck in between two extremes: obsessing about the optics of their meals or consuming food all day long without paying attention to the experience itself.

This isn't about nostalgia for some mythical past where everyone ate three square meals together or gathered around the fire to celebrate a successful hunt. Our ancestors had their own food challenges—extreme scarcity, limited variety, widespread famine, and life-threatening foodborne illness. But they also had something we've traded away: food that was embedded in shared culture, seasonal rhythm, and mindful satisfaction.

Looking Ahead: Why Traditional Diets Fail

By this point, you might be thinking, *Great, so I'm fighting biological hijacking AND cultural disruption. This feels hopeless.*

I understand that feeling. It can feel overwhelming when you realize how thoroughly Food 2.0 has rewired our food and eating environment, like discovering you've been playing a rigged game without knowing the rules were stacked against you.

But here's what I want you to know: Many people have found their way to a peaceful and purposeful relationship with food, even while living fully in the modern world. They haven't eliminated stress, sworn off convenience foods, or moved to a farm. They've simply learned to face these challenges and lead their Inner Eaters with care, creating islands of intention in the chaos of the modern food landscape.

To become a savvy consumer in an ultraprocessed world, you must understand why the traditional eating solutions you've been offered simply don't work. For decades, two dominant approaches have promised to solve our eating struggles: restrictive dieting and intuitive eating.

The first insists that you'll finally beat disease or get the body you want if you follow the right external rules—the perfect diet, the optimal meal timing, the correct macronutrient ratios. The second tells you to throw out all food rules and trust your body's natural wisdom to guide you.

Both approaches contain kernels of truth. Both have helped some people eat more intentionally. But both fall short when confronted with the realities of Food 2.0, often creating as many problems as they solve.

THREE

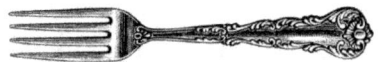

THE THREE DEAD-ENDS

WHY DIETS AND INTUITION CAN'T BEAT FOOD 2.0

"There comes a point where we need to stop just pulling people out of the river. We need to go upstream and find out why they're falling in."

ARCHBISHOP DESMOND TUTU

Before Sean ever experimented with tracking, fasting, or meal plans, he just . . . ate. Whatever was around. Whatever was easy. Some days, he threw together a decent breakfast. Other days, he grabbed a croissant and a latte at the shop on his morning walk. Lunch was whatever was fast, simple, and available.

Late-night pizza after a night out? No problem.

Bagels and coffee on the way to work? Standard.

A burrito the size of his forearm for lunch? Why not?

His metabolism seemed to keep up, and he stayed relatively lean without much effort. Food was just food. It was part of life, not something to be analyzed or worried about.

Then things started to change.

At first, it was subtle—constipation, sluggishness after meals, and brain fog that he couldn't shake. Then, his annual physical came back with numbers that made him pause. His LDL cholesterol was high. His blood sugar was creeping up. The doctor told him that, at this rate, he'd be diabetic in a year. That news hit him differently.

Sean had never seen himself as unhealthy. He had a few extra pounds around his midsection, love handles, sure, but he worked out regularly. He wasn't one of those guys who lived on junk food. And yet, here he was, starting to feel like his laissez-faire way of eating wasn't serving him anymore.

More than anything, he felt like he wasn't living up to his potential. He took pride in being disciplined in his career, finances, and relationships. But when it came to food, he was just winging it. The more he thought about it, the more it didn't sit right with him.

Sean began searching for a healthier way to eat, and his story illuminates why most of the common tactics people take to improve their eating fall short.

Path 1. Autopilot Eating: "Whatever, Whenever"

Autopilot eating is what happens when you let Food 2.0 call the shots. It is not really a path to eating better; it's more of an unconscious reaction to cravings, social cues, and whatever's most convenient. The danger is not realizing that you've outsourced all eating decisions to systems that don't have your health in mind.

(Remember the teens who all unknowingly were influenced to order the triple-dipped chicken.)

Autopilot eating feels easy because it is. You eat what's nearby, what others are eating, or what your emotions push you toward. For decades, this mode of eating worked for Sean. It was relatively thoughtless, frictionless, and—on the surface—functional. In a different culture or time period, this undiscerning eating style might have continued to work.

However, our hunter-gatherer instincts have been set loose in a supermarket the size of a football field, and for Sean, this meant his impulses could run free, eating with abandon.

Autopilot eating fails because when you eat unconsciously in a Food 2.0 environment, you won't just eat what your body needs; you will eat what the industry has designed for you to eat. This could lead you to experience the well-documented consequences of the *standard American diet* (SAD). There's a reason it's called a SAD diet; it's a fast track to chronic disease, worsening healthspan, and early death. The SAD is directly linked to rising rates of obesity, which affects over 42 percent of American adults.[1] It promotes Type 2 diabetes, where one in ten Americans are diagnosed, and many more are undiagnosed or clinically prediabetic.[2] And it advances cardiovascular disease, which is the leading cause of death in the United States.[3]

What's even sadder is that for many people, this way of eating isn't a choice; it's a socioeconomic reality. When fresh food costs more than processed food, and healthy options are out of reach, your Inner Eaters must adapt to survive. The Survival Eater becomes dominant, flagged by a price-sensitive Strategic Eater budgeting every penny. The Pleasure Eater takes whatever comfort it can get, and since Food 2.0 has mastered the art of cheap pleasure, that might mean a $6 fast-food value meal.[4]

Sean was lucky he wasn't financially strapped. He had the privilege of being able to shop at multiple grocery stores. He even had the time to cook if he wanted. Recognizing how the Food 2.0 environment threatened his health—over relying on deceptive marketing, cheap takeout meals, and convenience—prompted Sean to shift gears. He did what so many people do when they realize they're eating too many foods that promote insulin resistance, high cholesterol, and inflammation: He started a diet.

Path 2. Dieting:
"Follow the Rules, Stick to the Plan"

Sean woke up feeling motivated and ready to get back on track. If Path 1 involved surrendering to Food 2.0, Path 2 involved wrangling it under control.

He started with steel-cut oats and berries for breakfast. For lunch, it was grilled chicken, greens, and nuts. Everything was measured, planned, and tracked.

"This is the disciplined version of you that you've been waiting for," his Strategic Eater whispered in his ear.

The morning flew by. His inbox was under control, meetings were productive, and he was hitting his calorie goal for the day. In fact, the structure felt good. He liked having a plan, knowing exactly what to eat, and feeling like he was in control.

And it worked—at first.

The weight dropped, his digestion improved, and his energy felt more even. He seemed to have everything dialed in, and people took notice. The validation poured in: "Wow, you've lost some weight." "Your face looks so much younger." "How did you do it?" His friends asked for diet advice, and his doctor was impressed by his ability to lower his cholesterol.

THE ALLURE OF CONTROL

Dieting offers what autopilot eating never can: measurable results and a sense of order. It's a way to fight back against the status quo, to push back against Food 2.0's engineered consumption with clean rules and tight structure.

With a bit of validation, Sean went all in: No more mindless snacking. No more leaving it to chance. He had a plan, and for the first time, he thought, *I've cracked the code.*

His self-defined rules were:

- If food is the problem, control it.
- If weight is creeping up, cut calories.
- If sugar is addictive, eliminate it.
- If carbs/dairy/gluten/soy/seed oils (take your pick of vilified nutrients) are bad, don't eat them.

For Sean, giving his Strategic Eater sovereignty over his eating gave him a sense of control that felt intoxicating.

Walking past the office donuts? Easy. Saying no to late-night snacks? A badge of honor. Sean wasn't just eating better—he felt better than the people he knew who couldn't "control themselves" similarly.

But beneath the surface, things were starting to crack.

WHY DIETING FAILS

Sean started feeling anxious about social outings. What if there wouldn't be anything "clean" to eat when he got there? He felt uneasy when he had to travel, worrying about the lack of healthy food options and bringing back-up food "just in case." He second-guessed every indulgence. And the strangest thing? The more he controlled food, the more food controlled him.

What had started as a way to feel empowered around eating was now making him feel trapped. Why?

There are four reasons why dieting is a battle you can never fully win.

1. Diet culture thrives on the belief that your body is never good enough—that it's always in need of fixing, shrinking, or perfecting. But the pursuit of the "ideal body" isn't just exhausting; it keeps you locked in a cycle of self-judgment, making food choices from a place of fear of gaining weight, getting fat, or losing "the look."

2. Your Inner Eaters don't disappear; they rebel. The more you try to suppress your cravings, the louder they get. Restricting tasty food doesn't make your Pleasure Eater vanish; it just pushes it into the shadows, waiting for the right moment to strike back.

3. Willpower is exhaustible. You might be able to white-knuckle your way through a strict plan for a while, but the moment stress, fatigue, or strong emotions come into play, the discipline crumbles. Then what? Your Inner Eaters can only be wrangled into place for so long.

4. Diets create an all-or-nothing mindset. This black-and-white thinking fuels the binge–restrict cycle, erodes self-trust, and silences the curiosity needed to learn and adapt. It pits your Inner Eaters against each other, reinforcing shame and blame rather than the flexibility and nuance that real life demands.

When you're constantly chasing after some idealized way of eating or looking (which is unattainable for all but the most genetically gifted or uber-privileged), every meal becomes a test, every indulgence a failure, and your body becomes something to control rather than care for.

You follow rules, eliminate foods, chase outcomes, but you never address the deeper fears. You can control the menu, but without addressing the deeper programming—the unmet needs of your Inner Eaters—you end up reinforcing the very system crashes you hoped to escape. It's like trying to fix a computer by rearranging the desktop icons while the corrupted code keeps running in the background.

THE YO-YO DIETING TRAP: A BATTLE BETWEEN YOUR INNER EATERS

Diets create the illusion of being able to control your Inner Eaters, but in reality, they trigger a predictable battle, each one reacting to restriction in its own way. For instance:

- Your **Strategic Eater** takes absolute control. *I'm all in. I have a plan, and I'm sticking to it.* You commit with excitement, fueled by structure and discipline. Meal prepping, tracking macros, cutting out "bad" foods— it all feels empowering at first.

- Your **Pleasure Eater** starts simmering beneath the surface. At first, it plays along. But as cravings grow and your favorite foods stay off-limits, it starts whispering, *This sucks. Why can't we just enjoy food?* Every restriction only makes the temptation stronger.

- Your **Social Eater** feels isolated. Friends invite you out for dinner, but you're stuck calculating whether the menu fits your diet plan. Because you are avoiding social events that sound fun and interesting, you start feeling resentful when you have to "stay strong" while everyone else enjoys themselves. Ultimately, you're thinking, *Why can't I just eat like a normal person?*

- Your **Survival Eater** battles against starvation. It thinks your hunger is a sign of famine. It goes on high alert for anything it can get. When the opportunity for a snack or a few mindless bites arises, it seizes the moment, blowing up your plan and causing your Strategic Eater to rage in a fury.

This is precisely how the drama played out for Sean. The cravings for something other than chicken and broccoli began to creep in. The tracking started to feel exhausting. The occasional missed meal or off-plan snack started triggering guilt, frustration, and a feeling of failure.

And then came the all-or-nothing spiral. One moment of indulgence turned into "screw it mode." His Pleasure Eater and Survival Eater—suppressed for so long—came roaring back, throwing him into episodes of overeating.

Sean found himself trapped between control and rebellion, caught in the exhausting pendulum swing of letting one Inner Eater run the show.

WHY WILLPOWER ALWAYS FAILS

Inner harmony isn't won through suppression. It's earned through relationship. No matter how disciplined you are, if you're operating in a Food 2.0 world without awareness of your Inner Eaters, they will snap back into outdated patterns. In a battle between willpower and the Food 2.0 environment, Food 2.0 will always win.

This is exactly what the literature on dieting has so clearly revealed: Chronic dieting isn't just mentally exhausting; it's physiologically harmful in the following ways, among others.

- Eighty percent of dieters regain the weight they've shed (often more) within five years.[5]

- Chronic dieting slows metabolism, making weight loss harder over time.[6]

- There's an enormous psychological toll: anxiety, disordered eating, body dissatisfaction, increased food preoccupation, and so much more.[7]

Sean was tired of feeling like a failure every time he ate something "wrong." He knew he couldn't keep living like this. He needed a new approach—one that felt more natural, more freeing.

Path 3. Intuitive Eating: "Just Listen to Your Body"

Sean read about intuitive eating online and felt intrigued. No more counting calories. No more labeling foods as "good" or "bad." No more guilt over what you eat. Instead, you learn to trust your body, listen to your hunger and fullness cues, and eat in a way that feels natural. It sounded so appealing he threw away his kitchen scale and decided to give it a try.

The Promise of Food Freedom

At first, intuitive eating was a relief. Sean let go of the strict rules, and allowed himself to eat the foods he had avoided for so long. He gave himself unconditional permission to eat what he wanted, as the framework suggested. This was liberating.

For Sean and many of the other people I've coached who were looking to free themselves from years of food restriction, intuitive eating is a healing step—a way to recover from the damage caused by diet culture. Intuitive eating shifts the focus away from restriction and punishment and toward self-awareness and nourishment. Instead of battling against food and your hunger, it helps you learn to work with your body's signals, rebuilding a sense of trust that may have been eroded by years of dieting.

Pioneered by dieticians Evelyn Tribole and Elyse Resch, there are more than a hundred academic studies on intuitive eating, including a 2021 meta-analysis that found that the method is associated with lower rates of disordered eating, better psychological well-being, improved body image, and more stable weight regulation over time.[8]

At its core, intuitive eating teaches an important truth: The human body has immense wisdom. When you tune in to your body's signals rather than override them, you can cultivate more self-trust, which in turn, improves your relationship with food.

But there's a catch: In a Food 2.0 environment designed to confuse your body and overwhelm your mind, intuitive eating is not enough.

THE FOUR LIMITATIONS OF INTUITIVE EATING

The problem wasn't that Sean lacked intuition; it was that his intuition had been hijacked. Food 2.0 had actively reshaped the signals he was supposed to trust. What was he supposed to do if his body craved ultraprocessed foods that he knew left him feeling sluggish?

And what if his Pleasure Eater took the wheel and drove straight into a plate of cookies?

Also, what if his Social Eater made it too easy to say yes to pizza and happy hour every night because that's what everyone else was doing?

Here are four key limitations of intuitive eating as a complete approach to Food 2.0.

Limitation 1. Our hunger cues can be compromised. If you've spent years using food to manage stress or emotions, the difference between true hunger and emotional hunger becomes blurred. When eating becomes a habitual response to discomfort, your brain learns to associate food with relief, not just nourishment. This is especially true if you're on medication that suppresses or distorts your hunger and thirst. It's like trying to read a compass while standing next to a magnet: the signals are there, but they're being pulled in different directions.

Limitation 2. Food 2.0 disrupts our satiety. Highly processed foods trigger addictive-like responses, stimulating dopamine and opiate surges that drive overconsumption.[9] Your Pleasure Eater gets caught in a neurochemical feedback loop that keeps saying yes when your body should be saying, *"Enough."* Intuitive eating blames a diet mindset but overlooks the ways convenience stores, delivery apps, and engineered flavor profiles prevent your brain from saying *"I'm full. Stop eating."* It treats the modern food landscape as a trustworthy partner, but trusting Food 2.0 to regulate your appetite is like trusting a bartender to tell you when you've had enough.

Limitation 3. Social pressure overrides our internal cues. Your Social Eater doesn't just ask, *"Am I hungry?"* It asks, *"Will I feel left out if I don't eat?"* Intuition is always socially conditioned. What your dining partner is eating (or not eating) dramatically influence your food choices. You can't ignore what happens if your best friend passes you the bread basket and says, "You must try one of these. They're delicious."

Limitation 4. Moral neutrality obscures metabolic reality. A core tenet of intuitive eating is that all foods should be morally neutral, meaning no food is "good" or "bad." This is a crucial correction to diet culture's "better than thou" thinking. However, neutrality can become *nutritional blindness* when it comes to food quality and metabolic health. There is a significant difference between a banana and banana fosters, for example. Moral *neutrality* does mean metabolic *equivalency*. Moreover, permission to eat anything doesn't mean eating everything is wise—especially when Food 2.0 is manipulating you at the cellular level.

Intuitive eating practitioners often avoid discussing the health effects of different foods, fearing that it will sound like diet mentality and send people back into unhealthy restriction. However, people need to directly confront the real dangers of Food 2.0. This might mean making smart swaps or food upgrades in addition to adopting a morally neutral stance toward food.

Sean felt these limitations but didn't know what to do about it. He knew that some foods were more nourishing than others. But he also feared putting these foods off-limits and going back to a compulsive and strict mindset. He felt trapped in a false dichotomy: either full food freedom or full food control. What he was missing was an intelligent integration of these approaches that allowed him to choose well and eat well at the same time.

The Common Thread:
Why All Three Paths Fall Short

Each approach Sean tried made sense at the time and helped him improve his health and relationship with food. Dieting saved him from haphazard, autopilot eating by providing him with structure and education about nutrition. Intuitive eating helped him escape the rigidity and guilt of dieting while rebuilding body awareness.

But by themselves, all these paths were woefully incomplete, unable to manage with the laundry list of challenges that Food 2.0 presents.

This is where most people get stuck. They know they can't go back to autopilot eating, unless they're okay with a SAD ending. They know they can't go back to the all-or-nothing mindset of dieting, unless they're okay with feeling upset every time life doesn't go according to the plan. Lastly, they know they can't just rely on intuition to guide them through the maze of Food 2.0 supermarket shelves and social eating occasions.

The question is where to go next.

Beyond Right and Wrong:
The Garden of Eating 2.0

The Persian poet Rumi once wrote, "Somewhere beyond right and wrong, there is a garden. I'll meet you there." I'll extend the invitation: Somewhere beyond dieting and intuitive eating, there is a new way of eating. I'll meet you there.

Sean tried to fight Food 2.0 with willpower and intuition and failed because he was still playing with the wrong operating system. Hazel from the previous chapter felt dissatisfied with her eating because she couldn't see the ways Food 2.0 pulled her Inner Eaters in different directions. Both struggled because they were using outdated tools to navigate a system that requires an upgraded approach.

Looking Ahead:
Understanding the Voices Behind Your Choices

Understanding how Food 2.0 hijacks your biology and reshapes culture to maximize consumption is the first step toward real change. This awareness brings brutal honesty, and honesty is the fastest path to healing. The next step involves recognizing your Inner Eaters—Survival, Pleasure, Social, and Strategic—not as enemies to defeat, but as allies to understand, so you can blend intuitive wisdom with nutritional intelligence in service of the life you actually want.

PART II
THE INTERNAL PROGRAMMING

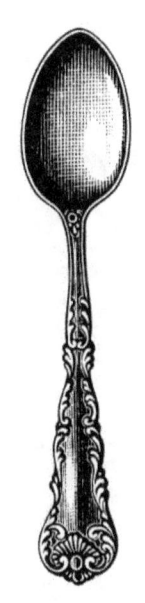

FOUR

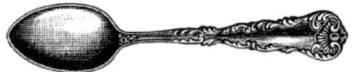

REVEALING YOUR CODE
THE FOUR KEYS TO FOOD FREEDOM

"Self-observation is necessary if we are to become free of our unthinking, mechanical reactions. If we do not observe ourselves, we cannot ever hope to be our own master. We will be like marionettes yanked by every impulse tugging on our strings."

DON RICHARD RISO

Standing in line at a crowded lunch spot, I leaned forward, squinting to read the specials board over the shoulders ahead of me. My brain had already begun placing bets on what I'd eat.

Lunch Special: Turkey, gruyere, avocado, tomato, green goddess dressing with microgreens on homemade sourdough.

The moment I saw the word *avocado* it triggered a thought: *good fats. Green goddess dressing* conjured creamy textures and good-looking Marvel heroines. *Gruyère* (although I could never pronounce it properly) evoked old, pleasant memories of melty cheese.

All of this happened in milliseconds, faster than conscious thought. My mind was processing and predicting lunch simultan-eously—the smell of bread, the sight of other people's sandwiches, and the rumble in my gut all contributed to the gestalt of the restaurant. My nervous system wasn't just experiencing the moment; it was getting emotionally invested in the outcome.

I glanced at the regular menu but felt overwhelmed. Too many options, too little time. My colleague picked up his meatball sub, buried in cheese and marinara. I could feel myself projecting my indecision onto his choice, classic internal confusion seeking external resolution.

Was he really going to eat the whole thing? Probably. But that wasn't really the point. The point was, I was already reeling inside.

In the past, I would have caved to the demands of the strongest urge. But this time, I maintained awareness of my Inner Eaters. I didn't argue, suppress, or overthink. I listened.

My Survival Eater spoke first. *"This is taking forever. You're hungry, and you've got a Zoom call in thirty minutes. Just order the ready-made sandwich."*

My Pleasure Eater chimed in, *"But they make amazing fried chicken here! Remember the crispy skin? The aioli?"*

My Strategic Eater fired back, *"You said no fried foods this week. Remember the heartburn? Go with the smoked salmon salad."*

My Social Eater scanned the room, then said, *"Everyone's getting the signature dish. Are you really going to be the only one with a salad?"*

I recognized each voice for what it was: a part of me with valuable perspective. But no voice had the whole story—that was for me to figure out. So, instead of letting any single part of me drive my decision, I stepped back and acknowledged:

- The urgency of my Survival Eater.

- The craving of my Pleasure Eater.

- The sensitivity of my Social Eater.

- The standards of my Strategic Eater.

Then, I took a breath. This was a new way of dealing with food stress, a new way of relating to myself, and I needed to be patient. For the first time, I was making space for contradiction without running away or immediately justifying one voice above all.

The CARE Model:
How I Made Peace with Food

That moment revealed the essence of upgrading our eating operating system: transcending and including the voices in our heads and impulses in our bodies to find the sweet spot where intuition meets wisdom, where food becomes fuel for the life we actually want.

The paradox is this: To make better food choices, you must first stop trying to make better food choices. Instead, turn your attention to your Inner Eaters—understanding what drives them and learning to consciously lead them toward harmony.

After years of food battles, I stopped trying to control my eating and started caring for the parts of myself behind those choices. That's when I developed the CARE model: a way to work *with* your Inner Eaters instead of *against* them, an approach grounded in four deceptively simple principles.

- **Curiosity.** Stop judging your hunger, preferences, or cravings and start getting curious. Ask them: *Why are you here, and what are you trying to tell me?*

- **Appreciation.** See that every part of you, even the ones that whine and beg, are there for a good reason, trying to help in their own way.

- **Responsibility.** Stop making excuses or giving away your power. Instead of blindly following the impulses of your Inner Eaters, take charge—set boundaries, shape environments, and build rhythms that support the eater you want to become.

- **Exploration.** Stop chasing perfect eating and start running experiments—*exploring* something new, *feeling* what works (and what doesn't), and *embodying* new ways of relating to your Inner Eaters.

Applied consistently, these four principles create something far deeper than a strategy; they become a way of being, a new inner code. Over time, CARE transforms eating from a struggle for control into a practice of conscious leadership and self-mastery with food.

What CARE Looked Like in Practice: (aka What I Actually Ordered)

So, what happened at that lunch? Let's walk through how I used the CARE model to avoid impulsive eating and make decisions that left me energized and satisfied instead of deprived or overstuffed.

C: CURIOSITY

Genuine curiosity means wanting to know the truth, not just the most convenient or familiar version of it. The most basic way to practice is by taking a pause. In that pause, curiosity interrupts automatic reactions and looks around for something new. Curiosity is all about *lingering*—something the breakneck speed of Food 2.0 culture rarely incentivizes.

At lunch, my Social Eater sensed everyone eating sandwiches and ran the script *"Sandwich equals fitting in."* This triggered the impulse to conform and order what I saw everyone else eating. Curiosity inserted a wedge into that impulse, letting me ask two questions.

1. *Who is actually eating right now?*

2. *Who is missing?*

I realized my Social Eater was the loudest voice, seeing this as an opportunity to connect with my colleague. It was saying, *"Maybe the meatball sub is a shortcut to rapport?"* But my Survival Eater was also present and frantic, having come straight from the gym on an empty stomach: *"Just eat. Get food fast. You have a call soon."*

Curiosity helped me name who was speaking, and also, who was silent. That second question—*Who's missing?* —was even more revealing than the first.

My Pleasure Eater, surprisingly, was quiet at first. What did I *really* want to eat? Was I too hungry to care? Did I even know my own preferences?

I began to notice a dual hunger: one in my stomach, the other in my mind. I had a hunger for mouth happiness, for that cheese-pull fantasy I hadn't named yet. And I had a raw, more primal hunger for essential nutrients and fuel.

I also noticed urgency. Not just to eat, but to *finish* eating. To get it over with and get on with my day.

Curiosity widened my awareness and allowed me to see that my anxiety was actually my Social Eater being apprehensive. My urgency was actually my Survival Eater feeling rushed. In both cases, I was no longer the feeling; I was the one witnessing them.

Psychologists call this ability to distinguish yourself (the subject) from your thoughts, feelings, and impulses (the objects) *subject-object differentiation*. It is a critical capacity in adult development, one that anyone can develop with consistent practice and the right support. Subject-object differentiation marks the shift from being run by your Inner Eaters to consciously leading them, allowing you to recognize that you are not the noise in your head, the hunger in your stomach, or the story you tell about it—you're the spacious capacity to hold it all. And in that space, choice returns.

CURIOSITY CREATES SPACE

Eating 1.0 says, "I'm starving. Eat now. Get rid of hunger."

Eating 2.0 asks, "Which Inner Eater is speaking—and what is it trying to tell me?"

Insight: Curiosity doesn't fix or force your Inner Eaters to change. It opens space inside the experience to create choices where there previously were none. Without curiosity, we stay trapped in judgment and reaction, never seeing the deeper patterns that control our eating.

A: Appreciation

Once I got curious, something softer opened up. I began to see that every part of me—yes, even those that used to drive me up the wall—was trying to help in its own way. I started using what psychologist Becky Kennedy, Ph.D., calls the *most generous interpretation* (MGI). The MGI begins with giving them the benefit of the doubt, assuming that my Inner Eaters are doing the best they can with the tools they have.[1] That doesn't mean they're always right. It means they're deserving of my respect and worth listening to.

So, rather than rolling my eyes at my Pleasure Eater's fried chicken fantasy, internally I acknowledged its wisdom. *Thank you for reminding me that meals should be enjoyable, not just functional.*

Rather than dismissing my Strategic Eater's push for a salad, I saw the intent behind the caution and acknowledged it. *You're not being a killjoy. You're trying to protect my future self from heartburn.*

This shift in tone matters. It changes the emotional environment of your nervous system from defensiveness to warmth. That warmth soothes the parts that feel upset or unheard. This may feel weird at the beginning, but that's only because most of us are far more practiced at beating ourselves up than listening kindly.

In an effort to practice MGI's, I made each part a quick internal promise.

- *Thanks, Survival Eater, food is on the way.*

- *Pleasure Eater, we'll get something that tastes really good.*

- *Social Eater, what I order won't make or break connection.*

- *Strategic Eater, we'll feel content and ready after this meal.*

This little act of mental appreciation of my different motives was a game changer. It may sound small—even silly—but something real happens when you name good intent—the noise quiets. The urgency softens. It was like each Inner Eater stopped shouting once they knew they'd been heard.

Appreciation is an emotional bridge between Curiosity and Responsibility. You can appreciate your Inner Eaters without agreeing with them. You don't have to like what they're saying to appreciate *why* they're saying it.

Appreciation sets the tenor for a relationship rooted in good intentions, mutual respect, and compassion. It says: *You belong here. I believe in you. We're on the same team.* That message creates psychological safety—the foundation for any lasting change.

APPRECIATION CALMS THE CHAOS

Eating 1.0 says: "I don't want to eat that. It's not okay."

Eating 2.0 says: "Every part of you is trying to help—even when it appears awkward or extreme."

Insight: When your Inner Eaters feel seen, validated, and appreciated, they calm down, allowing you to lead from a place of presence, not pressure.

R: Responsibility

Responsibility is often framed as an obligation or pressure to do something you'd rather not do—a heavy load to carry. But in Eating 2.0, we reclaim this word in its original form, defining it as the ability to respond.

Having response-*ability* means you're not stuck in reactivity. You're not being dragged around by whichever Inner Eater is shouting loudest. Instead, you're standing in the broader seat of conscious leadership—the one that can see all your parts, hear their concerns, and choose your next step with intention.

Responsibility makes the shift from "This is happening *to me*" to "I'm shaping what happens next."

Maybe you're thinking, *But sometimes I really don't feel like I have a choice. The craving hits. The temptation arises. I sit down to eat and the food is gone before I know it.*

We've all been there. But that's *exactly* the point of viewing response-ability as a muscle you can strengthen. You can't expect to be strong at something you've never trained. Nor do you wait to use it until it's perfect. When your capacity is high and the stakes are low, practice taking responsibility so you become familiar with what it feels like.

And even when you *do* "cave in" to your impulses, you still have response-ability after the fact. You can reflect on what happened and learn to respond differently next time. That, too, is conscious leadership.

For instance, if you keep eating after you're full, don't make yourself wrong. But you also can't complain about the stomach-ache later, as if it happened *to* you. That's not responsibility. It's victimhood.

The same principle applies on a larger scale. If you eat fast-food burgers and fries every day and then routine blood work shows elevated inflammation markers, you can't blame the lab or your genetics. That's victimhood.

You are responsible for taking care of your Inner Eaters, even if they're being hijacked by irresistible Food 2.0. This means acknowledging your role as conscious leader, noticing the consequences of your choices, and deciding how to act differently next time.

It is easy to fall into victim mode and perpetuate the same eating patterns that keep you stuck. There were plenty of times I lost or gave up my ability to respond, letting curiosity and appreciation fall to the wayside. Usually, I'd cave to whichever

Inner Eater was most afraid, eat impulsively, and then stew in regret about my fear-based choices. I wasn't responding, I was reacting, then resenting the aftermath.

Eating 2.0 responsibility means staying in relationship with your Inner Eaters long enough to make a choice that serves *more of you, more of the time.* Sometimes that means anticipating the tradeoffs *before* they bite you back. At other times, it means *reflecting* on a meal and deciding how you could have shown up as a better leader.

At that lunch counter, if I had gone with the salad:

- My **Strategic Eater** would've felt validated.

- My **Survival Eater** would've grumbled, *"This won't be enough."*

- My **Social Eater** might've worried that I'd look uptight.

- My **Pleasure Eater?** Rolling its eyes at the whole thing.

If I had gone with the meatball sub:

- My **Pleasure Eater** would've cheered.

- My **Strategic Eater** would've sounded the alarms: *"Too much fat, afternoon crash, regret loading . . ."*

- My **Social Eater?** Pleased as it matched my colleague's vibe.

- My **Survival Eater?** Happy for now, but probably paying the price two hours later.

No clear winner. No perfect choice. That's the point.

You might be thinking, *This cost-benefit analysis could go on forever. We'll never have all the details, all the consequences.* You're absolutely right. Analysis paralysis is a trap of the Strategic Eater.

In many ways, it's another form of fear in disguise—an evasion of responsibility.

Ultimately, you have to do your best to manage tradeoffs, giving every Inner Eater a seat at the table so no one has to throw a tantrum to be heard—and let that be enough for today.

At lunch, I found a dish that worked, more or less, for my whole Inner Eater family and took ownership of that choice 100 percent. I ordered the grilled chicken sandwich. Not fried, because that would sit heavy in my stomach, but not plain or bland. It came with fries, so I asked for a half portion with a side of greens, a compromise, not a copout. It was a responsible choice shaped by clarity and conscious leadership.

RESPONSE-ABILITY NOT RESTRICTION

Eating 1.0 says: "Why bother. There's no good choice. I'll just eat whatever."

Eating 2.0 says: "You made a choice. What can you learn from it?"

Insight: Responsibility isn't restriction. It's your ability to respond to your Inner Eaters—to lead them through tradeoffs, own the outcome, and build trust with yourself.

E: Exploration

Exploration is the pillar of possibility. It invites you to discover what else might work, especially when your default patterns feel rigid, unsatisfying, or self-defeating.

In neurocognitive terms, exploration is how we "rewire" the brain (forming new webs of connection between neurons).

Whenever you try something new, especially something that counters a well-worn pattern, you interrupt a neurological loop and introduce new information into your nervous system.

This pillar helps test the assumptions your Inner Eaters bring to the table. For instance, does fried food make you sluggish, or is that just something your Strategic Eater believes? Is a salad truly unsatisfying, or has your Survival Eater just never experienced one prepared in a way that is filling? Is leaving uneaten food on your plate unthinkable, or has your Social Eater been conditioned by years of childhood judgment?

These questions aren't answered in theory. They're answered through embodied data—sensed, tracked, tested, and tasted. That's how exploration works: not by thinking your way through eating, but by chewing your way to new choices.

Exploration also breaks binary thinking. Instead of choosing between healthy *or* indulgent, quick *or* quality, social *or* strategic, you begin discovering unexpected third options—ones that integrate more parts of you.

If you're science-minded, think like a researcher: tweak one variable and track the changes. For example, experiment with eating a bigger breakfast than normal and notice if your afternoon cravings shrink.

If you're more visual or creative, play with colors, plating, and textures. Try a new ingredient. Use a fancier dish. See what lights you up with joy. Exploration is an art and a science. Let your creativity lead and your scientific curiosity follow.

One caveat: Exploration works best when you're grounded. If you're stressed, have under slept, or are racing the clock, it's hard to hold the internal space needed to explore. Eating in a state of urgency will hijack your ability to respond and undermine any meaningful exploration.

But when you're regulated and your nervous system feels open and creative, you can approach eating as an *improvisational canvas*—a space to discover what nourishes you beyond the tried-and-true familiar eating experiences. This capacity to explore relies on true self-care and nervous system support. It depends on your ability to shift from threat mode (fight/flight/freeze) into play mode, where curiosity and new learning are most available.

So, how did I explore at lunch? I made two small shifts to my meal.

First, I asked for the delicious aioli on the side so my Pleasure Eater didn't go home empty-handed. That little splash of richness sent a signal: *You matter, too. Pleasure is important.* But it didn't steer the whole ship.

Second, I changed *how* I ate. I took a breath. I smelled the sandwich. I actually *looked* at the food—the black sesame seeds on the bun, the magenta-pickled onions tucked under the greens. Tiny moments of presence revealed textures and colors that I would have missed.

You know what? It tasted better.

I let my Pleasure Eater bring joy into the moment, and I invited my Survival Eater to relax. It didn't need to hoard or rush.

I asked my Strategic Eater to loosen its grip. We weren't solving the broken food system at this table. We were being thoughtful within reason.

Here's the beautiful part: I could eat peacefully with better awareness of my hunger and fullness. I didn't feel that familiar post-decision regret or anxiety. No more *I shouldn't be eating this*... thoughts plaguing me throughout the meal, and no ruminating later about calories.

The sandwich was good—not life-changing, but good—but it didn't need to be life-changing, because, for once, food wasn't carrying the weight of my Inner Eater's unmet needs. It was just lunch, satisfying, balanced, and conscious. That, my friend, is an Eating 2.0 upgrade.

EXPLORATION IS PERMISSION TO BE IMPERFECT

Eating 1.0 says: "I don't know what to eat" or "I must eat this."

Eating 2.0 says: "Try something new. Collect data. Learn and adapt."

Insight: You don't need perfect conditions, just the courage to try something different and observe what happens. Asking "What's possible?" opens doors that your Inner Eaters didn't even know existed.

Defining the Eater You Want to Become

When you develop a willingness to explore, there may be an implied objective or feeling like you need to get somewhere. For that, I have two suggestions.

One, don't set any objective. Just do something novel. You are traveling through an unfamiliar way of eating in order to learn about or familiarize yourself with it. You must avoid the trap of preconceived results to truly open yourself to discovery. The best bite in your life may be one you never planned or expected.

Two, ask this fundamental question: *What would the eater I want to become do right now—not perfectly, but confidently and courageously?* Let this be your exploration guide.

Your answer depends on your body, your story, your culture, and your desired future. Only you can define this vision, but here is a list of qualities that people consistently describe wanting in their relationship with food.

- Feeling calm and clearheaded when purchasing food
- Respecting hunger and fullness without letting either get out of control
- Making space for both pleasure and purpose in meals
- Eating with presence, not pressure, stress, or busyness
- Having time and patience to cook more
- Finding a balance between immediate gratification and long-term goals
- Being more consistent in aligning their daily choices with their values
- Being kind rather than critical when setbacks happen

TRY THIS:
REFLECT ON YOUR EATING ANCHORS

Take a moment to identify three valued traits or virtues that you want to bring to every meal. Examples might include:

Celebration	Trust	Mindfulness
Comfort	Growth	Peace
Connection	Health	Presence
Courage	Humanity	Relaxation
Craftsmanship	Integrity	Self-love
Creativity	Joy	Simplicity
Ecology	Justice	Spirituality
Gratitude	Kindness	Temperance

This list of valued traits is by no means exhaustive. It's a starting point for you to reflect on what really matters most in your life. Once you've identified a few values, write them down. These become eating anchors for you, as essential as a knife and fork. This way, the next time you sit down to eat, you've got your values as your compass and the four principles of the CARE model—curiosity, appreciation, responsibility, and exploration—to guide you.

Now, anytime you're stuck on an eating decision, you have upgraded inner programming to guide you. For example, if you're trying to decide whether to skip breakfast or eat something now before the days get busy, ask yourself, *What would bring more* (insert your chosen value) *to my Inner Eaters this moment?* If you're stuck between two options, explore how your chosen value would meet the moment. If you feel hungry but have just eaten, follow the CARE principles and explore what your chosen values would suggest in this situation.

What Upgrading Your Inner Programming Really Means

Without CARE, your Inner Eaters either operate unconsciously in the background or get treated like problems to eliminate. With CARE, they become parts of a symphony you are learning to conduct. This is what it looks like in the real world.

Not perfection, but presence. Instead of berating yourself for eating more chips than you need, you pause to notice your old programming in action. You promise to bring more awareness next time, discover what your Inner Eaters were seeking, and acknowledge that need with compassion.

Not domination, but direction. Rather than declaring "no carbs after 6 PM" and then demolishing a bag of chips at 11 PM, you recognize your Inner Eater's desire for late-night snacks and set loving boundaries, guiding them toward a snack you truly enjoy while honoring your nutritional goals.

Not control, but collaboration. When your Social Eater wants to eat out for the fourth night in a row this week and your Strategic Eater is worried about money and too many rich, heavy foods, you collaborate. You define expectations and areas of accountability by asking, *What are some reasonable ways forward*? Suggesting a friend come over for dinner? Cooking together? Grabbing an app out and then returning home?

The CARE model makes previously opaque eating moments more transparent and more relational. When food becomes a relationship you lead, rather than a battlefield where you merely survive, you build trust with your Inner Eaters, ultimately enhancing your ability to eat with presence, purpose, and peace.

Of course, there will be days when you feel completely lost and revert to old ways of eating. This is normal and expected. The most important skill to practice is relating to the tension you feel around food, not as a problem, but as a source of strength you haven't yet learned to harness.

This is a hard shift to make. I know because it took me years. I had assumed the way to eat better was to find the perfect plan that would finally stop the inner battle—to quiet the noise, to eliminate the stress, and to simply know what to eat. But here's what I discovered: Real intimacy and real growth require tension.

Your Survival Eater *should* want energy to keep you alive. Your Strategic Eater *should* push for long-term health. Your Pleasure Eater *should* want quick satisfaction. These aren't flaws in your system—they *are* the system. This inner tension is not a dysfunction. It's vitality.

All healthy systems, from forest ecosystems to family units, have tensions that ebb and flow. What keeps the system alive and resilient is not the absence of conflict, but how these tensions are managed, metabolized, and made meaningful.

It's the same inside you. Every Inner Eater brings a valid perspective, shaped by different needs, memories, and timescales. The friction between them generates insight. When you notice and navigate these tensions skillfully, you eat to meet your present needs, not to satisfy outdated cravings or rigid ideas of what "healthy" looks like.

When you don't know how to hold space for your tension, you try to suppress or escape it, and that's when eating goes off the rails. Upgrading your inner programming means letting the discomfort be there, without letting it drive. CARE doesn't remove the tension—it helps you meet it skillfully, so it energizes your choices instead of triggering a power struggle. Over time, the tension bothers you less. It's not such a big deal to simultaneously want different things or feel two ways about food. The spaciousness and freedom *to simply eat* emerge as a result of embracing this inner complexity, rather than forcing it to go away.

CARE-ful Eating vs. "Clean" Eating

Let me be clear: I'm not saying the grilled chicken sandwich was the "right" lunch choice or the fried chicken was "wrong." That would be finite Eating 1.0 thinking. Eating 2.0 is about responsiveness, context, and consequence.

When you upgrade your eating operating system, the illusion of a *single right choice* disappears. With your wider and wiser awareness, you see there's only your best relationship with the moment you're in. Let me explain how this concept would apply to my lunch.

If I had eaten something different for breakfast, had dinner plans that night, skipped the gym that morning, or felt a little more adventurous, my Inner Eaters would be giving me different feedback that might lead to different choices. Maybe I would've experimented with the fried chicken to test my Strategic Eater's assumption that it results in heartburn or sluggishness. Perhaps I would have tried the salad to challenge my Survival Eater's fear that it won't be satisfying. Or maybe I could have done something that honors both: a salad with fried chicken on top!

The point isn't to "eat clean." It's to eat with clarity, to make conscious choices that reflect your whole system: survival biology, personal preferences, social pressures, and personal and planetary goals. As a conscious participant in the infinite game of nourishment, you begin to think in terms of play, not punishment, creativity, not compliance. This requires addressing how Food 2.0 leads your Inner Eaters to extremes. It also requires considering the unintended consequences of changing one part of your eating without honoring the full range of voices within you.

And if you don't manage the challenges of Food 2.0 or take care of your Inner Eaters? No shame. You're planting seeds of change.

The point is this: You are not wrong for eating the way you currently do.

This bears repeating. You are not wrong, lesser, or in any way unworthy for eating the way you do. Until you accept this truth deep in your bones, do not proceed.

Accepting yourself as you are now doesn't mean you are happy with your eating. Nor does it mean your current diet is helping you be healthy. You would not be reading this book if you didn't believe there are more satisfying, balanced, and intentional ways to eat. But at the fundamental level, your eating is not broken. Even if you've been through years of struggle, you are always only one meal away from making new choices. So, don't waste energy ruminating over lost time. Learn from the past and move forward compassionately and courageously.

Looking Ahead:
Getting to Know Your Inner Eaters

Now that you understand the CARE model, it's critical to know your Inner Eaters deeply, like dear friends. Otherwise, you're stuck with surface-level understanding that leads to lazy labels, such as:

- The **Survival Eater** is "impulsive."
- The **Pleasure Eater** is "indulgent."
- The **Social Eater** is "people pleasing."
- The **Strategic Eater** is "controlling"

These crude stereotypes only capture the negative aspects of your Inner Eaters when they're forced into maladaptive roles, dysregulated by Food 2.0. But as you'll discover, behind each reactive form of these parts lies incredible wisdom, and leveraging their wisdom is the springboard to becoming the eater you want to be.

In the coming chapters, we'll explore each Inner Eater in depth so you can learn where each Inner Eater comes from; how they protect you or sometimes sabotage you; how to recognize their voice in real time; and most importantly, how to CARE for them to reclaim your power.

Let's start with the one who shows up when life gets hectic, hunger hits hard, and there's no time to think: Your Survival Eater.

CARE QUESTIONS

CARE is your conscious leadership toolkit. Use it anytime you feel torn, triggered, or tempted to check out around food; go through the CARE questions.

1. C: *Who's driving this eating? Who's missing?*

2. A: *What's their positive intent?*

3. R: *What tradeoff or consequences will I 100 percent own?*

4. E: *What haven't I tried yet?*

Try bringing CARE to one eating moment today and see what happens. You might be surprised what emerges through conscious care rather than brute force.

FIVE

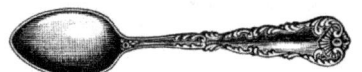

YOUR SURVIVAL EATER

THE RELENTLESS GUARDIAN WHO FEARS GOING HUNGRY

"It is not accidental that all phenomena of human life are dominated by the search for daily bread."

IVAN PAVLOV

"Just need some water," I mumble, reaching for the glass on the bedside table. I see my phone light up. It's 7:42 AM. My alarm didn't go off.

Shit.

My morning class at Harvard starts in forty-eight minutes, and I planned on biking to campus. The issue? I would not be another tired student sitting in a lecture hall; *I was supposed to be delivering the lecture.*

I rush through my morning routine, frantically trying to make up for lost time. I haphazardly get dressed and search for my laptop.

123

Phone, check. Jacket, check. Peace of mind? Gone. The whole thing feels chaotic.

As I'm about to dash out the door, my stomach growls. I haven't eaten, and I know that once class starts, it will be hours before I get another chance. I start scanning the kitchen for something—anything—that requires zero preparation and can be consumed in seconds. The bar in my bag. The apple on the counter. Whatever gets calories into my body with minimal disruption.

This isn't laziness. This is survival.

Who comes to the rescue? My Survival Eater! It doesn't care about culinary perfection or nutritional optimization. It has one job: keep me fed with the least possible expenditure of time, effort, and mental bandwidth. In a world of nonstop demands, jam-packed schedules, and borrowed energy, this part is working overtime.

Evolutionary Origins: Wired for Survival

Your Survival Eater is your practical protector—the part of you that prioritizes speed, ease, and efficiency when it comes to food. It evolved in a world where food was unpredictable and energy conservation was critical to survival. Our ancestors couldn't afford to waste precious calories on inefficient food acquisition, so every food choice answered a simple question: "Is the energy I'll gain worth the energy I'll expend to get it?"

This calculus is hardwired into our biology. Our brain, which consumes about 20 percent of our energy despite being only 2 percent of our body weight, is constantly looking for efficiency shortcuts. It's why we opt for the easiest path across a parking lot (even at the gym!), why we develop habits that require less thinking, and why, when tired, overwhelmed, or rushed, we reach for whatever food requires the least effort.

This survival instinct is still alive and well today. When Sean grabbed pizza between meetings (remember his story from Chapter 3) he wasn't being gluttonous; his Survival Eater was performing triage, keeping him fueled during a relentless workday.

This part of you operates on a straightforward premise: Fed is better than perfect. That's why protein bars exist. That's why canned soup is a pantry staple. That's why cold pizza is the ultimate "whatever's available" food. Your Survival Eater understands that safe, reliable food is the answer when energy is limited, whether due to stress, illness, overwork, or the need to handle competing responsibilities. Ever eaten a sad, unheated plate of leftovers while standing in your kitchen, staring blankly into space? Congratulations, you've met your Survival Eater.

Recognizing Your Survival Eater's Voice

You Survival Eater speaks the language of sensation, such as stomach growls, pressure, emptiness, gnawing, and rumbles. Its voice accompanies the urge to eat when feeling depleted or the urge to eat when food is staring at you across the table. This Inner Eater goes on high alert when people start talking about food, or your nose catches a faint whiff of something delicious.

Over time, these sensations and impulses become recognized as the message *"You're hungry"* or *"Just eat something. Anything."* In truth, these are after-the-fact justifications for what your body already knows: Survival is at stake; it's time to refuel before resources run out.

The difficult part is that the English language doesn't have great words and phrases for talking about the voice of your Survival Eater. *Hunger* or *gut feeling* are fine, but they are too broad and ambiguous to truly convey the felt experience of wanting to eat or needing food. You may say, "I feel ravenous" or "I have a voracious appetite," but these remarks only point to the famished side of your Survival Eater.

On the other end, there's "I'm stuffed" or "uncomfortably full." Yet none of these words capture the rich, dynamic interplay of signals your body sends—stomach stretch receptors, hormonal feedback, vagal tone, glucose levels, the subtle tugs of anticipation or aversion.

Your Survival Eater is constantly speaking a language of need, safety, and energy balance, yet we have only crude approximations to describe these feelings. Moreover, Food 2.0 diverts our attention elsewhere, leaving your Survival Eater to shout, *"Pay attention to me,"* even when your brain is busy with a thousand other things. It speaks a language older than words, an embodied reminder that you are an animal before you are anything else. Pretend you don't hear it, and it'll come back as a primal demand you can't negotiate with.

If you're like most people, then your Survival Eater gets louder:

- During prolonged periods of not eating.
- During high-stress periods.
- When you have overbooked your schedule and don't have time to eat.
- In times of transition, such as while moving, starting a new job, or having a new baby.
- When you're experiencing physical illness or exhaustion.
- If you're under financial strain and need to make difficult decisions about how much food you can afford.
- When you have overwhelming responsibility for others' needs.

- During travel that disrupts eating routines or limits access to familiar foods.

These are precisely the circumstances when survival-based eating becomes more important. Your Survival Eater assesses that your resources are limited and may drive you to the simplest, most convenient eating options. It knows that overthinking food when life demands efficiency may be costing you more than it's worth.

TRY THIS:
SELF-ASSESS

Think about your internal dialogue around food. When do you feel your Survival Eater most strongly? What circumstances amplify its urgency?

The Wisdom of Your Survival Eater

If you've ever started a diet, felt motivated for a week, and then watched it collapse the moment life got stressful, you've already met your Survival Eater. It doesn't care that you're "supposed" to avoid refined carbohydrates or stop eating late at night. It will drive you to eat whatever's closest and easiest because you are an animal trying to make it to tomorrow.

For example:

- Your blood sugar is dipping, and there's a box of candy on the shelf—that's why it's called a LifeSaver, isn't it?

- You've been awake for eighteen hours and are feeling depleted. Let's see what's in the fridge.

127

- You're running short on time and feeling hungry. What about that gas station hot dog on the way home?

- You scan the menu feeling ravenous, as if you're starving. What dish will give you the biggest bang for your buck?

Your Survival Eater is primarily concerned with keeping your bodily system running. It conserves energy, prioritizes calories, and minimizes the chances of genuine starvation. If your eating doesn't respect these biological facts, your best intentions will get overridden.

When your Survival Eater is balanced, its pragmatic and resourceful energy enables you to:

- **Stay fueled when life is busy.** A quick smoothie, a handful of nuts, or a simple meal to keep you going when time is tight.

- **Make eating simple.** It cuts through decision fatigue—no elaborate meal plans, no endless culinary customizations. Good enough is good enough.

- **Adapt on the fly.** When you're traveling, at an airport, or on a road trip, this Inner Eater helps you to keep moving.

Consider Hazel from Chapter 2, juggling her marketing career with raising a young child. Her Survival Eater was operating under the assumptions of limited time and energy. In its own way, this part was trying to protect her—making sure she didn't skip meals entirely and that she could keep going through long, demanding days. Its reliance on premade meals and ready-to-eat snacks reflected a reasonable belief: *You can't pour from an empty cup, so fill it however you can.*

The Shadow Side of the Survival Eater: When Convenience Becomes Compulsion

Your Survival Eater is particularly vulnerable to exploitation by the endless eating of Food 2.0. It never evolved to navigate a world of on-demand delivery, drive-through windows, or the enchantment of breakroom donuts. As discussed in Part I, the food industry has mastered making unhealthy choices cheap and convenient while positioning more nourishing options as expensive and time consuming.

If your days heavily rely on premade meals, energy drinks, and whatever is closest to your laptop, your Survival Eater is following the path of least resistance. This is not necessarily an issue, but without awareness, it is easy for the food industry's goals to overrule your own.

Here are some common ways in which overreliance on your Survival Eater can lead you astray.

- **It becomes chronically rushed,** giving you the impression that time and energy are limited.

- **It fails to adapt as circumstances change,** maintaining "survival mode" eating patterns even when you have more resources available.

- **It becomes entangled with physical coping,** making eating a way to release or distract yourself from pain.

- **It gets dysregulated by Food 2.0,** creating cravings and crashes, blunting satiety, and disrupting hormonal balance.

- **It minimizes eating pleasure,** turning meals into something to "get through" rather than something to stop and enjoy.

Notice if you habitually sacrifice quality for speed, or talk yourself out of the nutritionally better, but slightly more demanding eating option. This might be a sign your Survival Eater is strong-arming you to make it the sole voice dictating all your food choices.

The Fears That Drive Your Survival Eater

Beneath its practical facade, your Survival Eater harbors deeper fears than simply running out of time or energy. These fundamental anxieties shape its behavior in ways you might not recognize.

Fear of uncertainty. Your Survival Eater gravitates toward familiar foods, smells, and textures because the unknown represents risk. New foods might be spoiled, contain allergens, or upset your digestive system. That is why this part of you chooses what it knows will keep you alive rather than taking a chance on eating something unfamiliar.

Fear of physical harm. Your Survival Eater is hypervigilant about safety, both in terms of food and your body. Because it evolved from the prehistoric maxim "Eat now or be eaten," it's operating under the belief that danger might strike at any time, and eating itself makes one vulnerable to attack. The result is a basic urge that says, *"Don't linger. Eat quickly and move on."*

Fear of death. Perhaps the most powerful fear is that you might not get another chance to eat if you don't eat now. This fear of death, whether from actual past experiences of food insecurity or the millennia of food scarcity baked into our genes, fuels opportunistic and impulsive eating. It is why we are quick to avoid anything that might resemble famine. (*That will never be enough. I'll still be hungry!*) This is also why we prefer calorie-dense, quick-energy foods, especially when we're stressed or tired.

Once you start recognizing your Survival Eater's fears, you'll also notice how Food 2.0 marketing messages mimic and amplify these exact thoughts.

- "Grab and go!" appeals to its desire to get in, get fed, and get out
- "Hungry? Why wait?" targets its fear of deprivation
- "Buy one, get one free" exploits its scarcity mindset

The food industry has weaponized your Survival Eater's protective instincts, turning them against your long-term well-being.

Your Survival Eater's Personal History

Your personal history, everything from living with food scarcity to a lifestyle with relentless time pressure, influences how dominant your Survival Eater becomes. Let me share a few stories to help illustrate how this Inner Eater takes shape and when its adaptive instincts become maladaptive eating habits.

FROM SCARCITY TO SAVORING: BREAKING OUT OF DEFAULT SURVIVAL MODE

Eli grew up in a house with four brothers, where mealtimes were a feeding frenzy: Get what you can, eat it fast, and hope for seconds. This food insecurity hyperactivated his Survival Eater, making him extraordinarily sensitive to food cues—he could detect the sound of someone opening the refrigerator from across the house.

While these instincts were helpful in childhood, as an adult with financial security, he still found himself racing to finish meals, attending events for free food, and grabbing snacks just because they were available. His Survival Eater wasn't there to dine; it was there to feed.

I experienced something similar during the first few months of parenthood. The sleep-deprived chaos of caring for a newborn left little time to eat, giving my Survival Eater the perfect opportunity to take control. I shoveled food into my mouth whenever possible—while cleaning bottle parts, restocking diapers, and supporting my postpartum wife. Like Eli, I wasn't really experiencing the food. I was there to feed.

The transformation came when we both realized our Survival Eaters had claimed territory beyond their proper domain. What started as necessary adaptations had become our default relationship with food, even when circumstances no longer demanded it.

For Eli, the wake-up call came during his honeymoon when his wife noticed he'd finished an elaborate dinner in under four minutes. "When she asked if I'd even tasted it, I couldn't answer," he shared. "I literally couldn't remember what I'd eaten."

For me, it was asking myself: *When did eating become such an afterthought, just another task to check off?* Once upon a time, food had been a source of pleasure and connection for me. Now, in the new baby fog, it was merely fuel, consumed with mechanical efficiency.

We both learned the same crucial lesson: Any learned eating pattern can be unlearned. How we ate wasn't some immutable facet of our personalities; it was an adaptation of our Inner Eaters to our circumstances. What came next was teaching our Survival Eaters to show up differently, not through rigid rules or impossible standards, but through small moments of caring awareness and choice.

Eli began by setting a timer during meals—just five minutes at first, extending the experience slightly beyond his comfort zone. This was Eli's way of taking responsibility for the hurried energy his Survival Eater brought to meals and exploring new ways of containing that energy. "I had to convince this part of me that the famine was over," he explained. "It wasn't easy. For thirty years, that part kept me alive by grabbing and consuming everything as quickly as possible."

The breakthrough came when Eli was alone at a buffet while traveling for work. "All my old triggers were there—unlimited food, no one watching, and old anxieties bubbling up. But for the first time, I could hear my other Inner Eaters too: the parts that wanted to select food deliberately, taste what I was eating, and relax into my dining experience."

That day, Eli didn't override his Survival Eater, he partnered with it. He acknowledged its fears, honored its protective intentions, and gently guided it toward a new possibility: That he could take his time to eat because the food was not going to run out.

THE HYPERVIGILANT RESPONSE: "HUNGRY? WHY WAIT!"

Your Survival Eater might rush to grab a snack at the first stomach grumble, not because it's necessary, but because it's become allergic to even the faintest signs of hunger. This isn't irrational or uncommon. We live in a world where productivity demands leave little room for physical discomfort, and food marketing frames hunger as something to eliminate immediately.[1] Who wants a mild ache in the stomach to disrupt a work call or distract from time with family? If hunger is a solvable problem, then solve it. It's like adjusting the air-conditioning if you're feeling too hot. Modern life has made these nuisances a relic of the past.

The question then becomes: How much hunger can you tolerate? If the answer is zero, then you're setting yourself up for a very narrow bandwidth of what feels comfortable. You might even eat because *you fear you might get hungry*, preemptively trying to keep your tank from hitting empty. This hypervigilant approach to hunger makes sense in a world of food scarcity, but less so when food is endless, effortless, and irresistible.

THE DISCONNECTED RESPONSE: "TOO BUSY TO BE HUNGRY"

Opposite to hypervigilance is disconnection. Your Survival Eater might ignore hunger signals entirely when work pressure consistently takes precedence over mealtimes, or when chronic stress keeps your body in fight-or-flight mode. Coffee and stimulants can also disrupt your Survival Eater. This masks hunger signals, creating extreme cycles where hunger builds unnoticed, then your Survival Eater reacts by grabbing whatever is fastest rather than most nourishing. Danny, the CEO of a large pet supply company and a former client, illustrates the pitfalls of a disconnected Survival Eater.

As CEO, he lived by one rule: "The machine never stops." His body was merely a vehicle for ambition. His Survival Eater was the only Inner Eater he could access, and it ruled his life—office coffee and pastries for breakfast, trays of sandwiches in the boardroom for lunch, energy drinks for afternoon slumps, evening takeout while reviewing financials, and alcohol to wind down.

For Danny, the thought of pausing to actually think about what he ate felt like a luxury he couldn't afford. That was until his diet and nonstop lifestyle made his arthritis so bad it became difficult to walk. What terrified him most wasn't the pain but his inability to envision another way. His convenience-based eating pattern had become so ingrained that even in crisis, cooking a meal or researching anti-inflammatory foods seemed as impossible as climbing Everest. He unconsciously allowed his Survival Eater to operate without balance or leadership. Regaining his health required that he upgrade internal programming, balancing his Survival Eater's Stone Age instincts with the food realities of a modern executive.

Reconnecting with Your Body's Signals

Your body keeps the score in the survival game. Therefore, you need to reestablish a connection with your body's hunger and fullness signals to lead your Survival Eater effectively. This doesn't mean becoming hyper attuned to every sensation (there's a way to overdo everything), but it does entail developing a more attentive and nuanced relationship with your bodily cues.

The next time you notice yourself reaching for food, pause to inquire: *How do I know I'm actually hungry? What am I feeling right now?*

Physical hunger signals might include:

- Pangs in your stomach that slowly grow in intensity.

- Predictable hunger patterns at certain times.

- Energy depletion or weakness.

- Grumpiness (the famous "hanger").

- An indiscriminate desire to eat anything available.

- Heightened awareness of food-related sensory cues.

This list isn't exhaustive. Everyone experiences hunger uniquely, and your own signals may change from day to day. The critical part is directing your attention inward. Where do you experience hunger first? Can you locate it precisely in your body?

The challenge is that your Survival Eater tends to categorize many sensations as hunger, including thirst, boredom, anxiety, or fatigue. If you've conditioned it to believe eating is the fastest path to relief from these sensations, it will default to food regardless of the root cause. The way forward is to slowly build your capacity to notice sensation as nothing more than energy in your body. You can begin to distinguish between types of hunger and degrees of urgency. With time, you can reprogram your Survival Eater to treat hunger not as a reflex to eat, but information deserving your deeper attention.

Teaching Your Survival Eater about Fullness

In its rush to resolve hunger quickly, your Survival Eater often overshoots the point of satisfaction, reaching an uncomfortable level of fullness. It's your job to help it recognize the difference between quieting hunger and reaching fullness. Despite common misperception, the two are not the same. The easiest way to start is by taking deliberate pauses during meals to assess:

- *Am I paying attention to sensations of fullness or just eating until the food is gone?*

- *Where do I first experience fullness? How does this shift as the meal continues?*

- *If I stopped eating now, would I be satisfied? How do I know I need more?*

Your Survival Eater benefits from a mindful approach, helping it feel safe enough to slow down. Even a five-second pause to notice your current physical state can help it develop a more accurate gauge of hunger and fullness.

Leading Your Survival Eater Wisely

Your Survival Eater may have developed some unhelpful habits adapting to the Food 2.0 world. Here are some practical first steps to transform your relationship with this primal part of yourself and provide conscious leadership.

CURIOSITY:
UNDERSTANDING YOUR SURVIVAL EATER'S PATTERNS

I used to think my grab-and-go eating habits were just poor planning. (To be fair, that was still an important missing piece.) Then I got curious about what feelings were driving my food choices, and I discovered something fascinating: My Survival Eater took control at two predictable times—frantic weekday mornings and back-to-back afternoon meetings. During these windows, every food choice was filtered through one question: "What's least disruptive to my schedule?" Once I recognized this pattern, I could use the other CARE principles to create better options that still honored my time constraints.

ONE PRACTICE:
THE SURVIVAL TRIGGER MAP

Carry a small notecard or use a notes app on your phone for three days. Each time you eat, pause for thirty seconds to record:

1. The time of day.
2. Your hunger level on a scale of 1–10.
3. The main feeling present (rushed, tired, hungry, overwhelmed, and so on).
4. Your current constraints. Is it time? Energy? Decision fatigue? Something else?

Don't judge what you discover—simply collect the data. At the end of three days, look for patterns. Most people find their Survival Eater has specific activation points, like the 3 PM energy crash, the morning stomach grumble, or when traveling or commuting.

APPRECIATION:
HONORING YOUR SURVIVAL EATER'S INTENT

Behind every grab-and-go meal is sophisticated resource management. Thank your Survival Eater for keeping you functioning during insane deadlines, finals week, new parenthood, or that brutal stretch of travel. It's handling food logistics so your higher brain can focus on putting out fires.

ONE PRACTICE:
THE DAILY ACKNOWLEDGMENT

The next time you feel yourself reaching for the fastest food option available, place your hand on your shoulder (like you would when comforting a friend) and say: *Thank you for keeping me going. I see how hard you work to manage my energy and prevent hunger.*

Take one full breath and then reassure this part of your partnership and guidance. *This isn't a crisis. A little hunger is okay. We can eat later if needed. I promise we won't starve. Trust me.*

Many of my coaching clients report that when their Survival

Eater feels genuinely seen for its protective role, the frantic "anything will do" energy begins to calm. This opens the door for conscious leadership rather than reaction.

RESPONSIBILITY:
CREATING STRUCTURE FOR SUCCESS

Responsibility isn't about swearing off vending machines or banning fast food forever. It's about taking ownership of the Food 2.0 system your Survival Eater operates in, especially in predictable, high-stress environments.

Now that you understand this part of you gets triggered by energy dips, food marketing, and back-to-back obligations, you can create conditions where making better choices is easier.

ONE PRACTICE:
THE ENVIRONMENT UPGRADE

Choose one location where your Survival Eater frequently takes control—perhaps your workplace, car, or kitchen. For this one location, implement the following three changes.

- Notice how food labels speak to your Survival Eater: What promises does the marketing make about speed, convenience, or energy?
- Remove a Food 2.0 item that manipulates your Survival Eater into unnecessary hurry and worry.
- Add one new food option that doesn't exacerbate survival-based thinking.

Alex, a former client, applied the environmental upgrade practice to his workplace eating. On the days when he was in back-to-back meetings—which, honestly, was almost every day—he would usually run to the vending machine and grab a bag of pretzels or Cheetos instead of having a full lunch. This snack became his Survival Eater's go-to energy source. But what started as a protective way to ward off hunger, became hijacked by Food 2.0's engineered cravings.

"I was spending like twenty-five dollars a week on vending machine snacks," Alex told me, "and I'd feel terrible afterward—not just physically, but because I knew I was smarter than this." But when Alex's afternoon energy crash hit during a difficult work session, his brain just went straight to *"Need salt and crunch NOW."*

Alex began to recognize how his Survival Eater was totally in control, reacting to the fear of deprivation. But instead of letting this part blindly lead him to the vending machine, Alex took responsible leadership by changing his environment.

His simple upgrade: He started bringing a small container of mixed nuts in his laptop bag and a piece of fruit from home. "The key was making it just as convenient as the vending machine," he explained. "I kept the snacks right next to my laptop charger, so I'd see them every time I packed my bag." It wasn't that the nuts were any less fatty or caloric than the Cheetos, but they weren't as addictive, and he felt much better after eating them.

That's what responsibility looks like: taking care of your Survival Eater's needs without caving in to its cries. The opportunity is to curate the eating options your Survival Eater will default to because better options equal better decisions.

EXPLORATION:
FINDING YOUR SURVIVAL SWEET SPOT

If *responsibility* prepares the field, *exploration* shifts the pattern. It is how you teach your Survival Eater what's possible when it doesn't act alone, inviting it to collaborate with the rest of your inner team.

Laura, a busy parent with two teenagers, assumed ordering takeout was the easiest way to get fed. However, she discovered through the practice of exploration that her Survival Eater wasn't necessarily demanding delivery food. It was feeling depleted and asking for relief from decision fatigue. "I didn't need to spend energy choosing what to eat," she said. "I needed simple, reliable options that were already within reach."

By giving her Survival Eater immediate, low-effort satis-faction—whether a few precooked staples in the fridge or a go-to grocery shortcut—she avoided the overwhelm of long menus and endless choices. Her Strategic Eater helped her reduce friction without adding effort, keeping her nourished and preventing reactive, impulsive eating.

PRACTICE:
ONE-MINUTE INTEGRATION

This week, choose one moment when your Survival Eater is driving your decisions: a rushed lunch between calls, snacks on the go, or dinner when you're too tired to cook.

Instead of hurrying ahead, stay with your experience and ask:

- *What would bring a touch of pleasure to this moment?*
  (Pleasure Eater)

- *What simple upgrade would support my longer-term health?* (Strategic Eater)

- *How can I move from isolation to connection—even just with myself?* (Social Eater)

Then act on a tiny shift. For example:

- Plate your food instead of eating from the container.

- Sit somewhere you can actually notice your food.

- Pause before eating to remember, *I'm taking care of myself right now. I am allowed to eat, not just feed.*

After this moment of experimentation, reflect on these questions.

- *What did I learn about what my Survival Eater truly needs versus what it habitually chooses?*

- *How did the quality of my eating experience change when I brought leadership and integration, even if my food choices remained the same?*

- *What specific shifts worked best for me?*

Looking Ahead: From Survival to Pleasure

Your Survival Eater evolved to keep you alive in a world of scarcity, but if you're lucky enough to have an abundance of food options, there's a good chance you're not in survival mode anymore (at least not all the time). The issue is that modern life can be so fast-paced, overstimulating, and hyperconnected that your nervous system *feels* like everything is a matter of survival. This misperception keep your Survival Eater making panic-based decisions when you don't really need to.

The reward of consciously caring for your Survival Eater is greater trust in yourself. When you acknowledge, respect, and give your Survival Eater direction, you gain a reliable team member—a pragmatic protector helping you navigate real-world constraints.

As you become more skilled at recognizing and collaborating with your Survival Eater, you might notice something surprising: Many of the choices you thought were yours are actually reactions to Food 2.0's marketing. When your Survival Eater feels less manipulated and more supported, it creates space for eating to be a source of pleasure, not just pragmatics. This is where we will go in our next chapter.

In the next chapter, you'll meet your Pleasure Eater—the part that seeks joy, satisfaction, and sensory delight in food. While it might seem at odds with your convenience-minded Survival Eater, these two members of your Inner Eater family can work together to turn eating into a source of practical enjoyment.

SIX

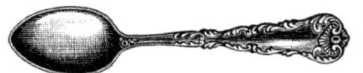

YOUR PLEASURE EATER
THE JOY SEEKER WHO WANTS ANOTHER BITE

"To know what you prefer, instead of humbly saying Amen to what the world tells you you ought to prefer, is to have kept your soul alive."

ROBERT LOUIS STEVENSON

"**F**ive down. Eleven to go," I excitedly said to my wife across the table. We were in the midst of a sixteen-course tasting menu at one of Lima's finest restaurants. This wasn't vacation—this was a pilgrimage. My wife and I had journeyed to Peru to experience culinary artistry. We wanted to eat the creations of chefs whose restaurants ranked among the world's best.

In the courtyard of a colonial mansion-turned-restaurant, a server presented a scallop seared to perfection, nestled in its shell atop a dramatic base. "Number six," I proclaimed, grinning like a kid who's just mastered numbers and counting.

The aroma of warm, melting cheese wafted toward me. I watched my wife's expression transform with her first bite, a look of pure satisfaction as she chewed. I leaned in for my turn.

As that scallop morsel melted on my tongue, a perfect mix of delicate and creamy, a revelation struck: This transcendent moment differed from most of my daily bites. It wasn't just that the food was exquisite. It was that I was fully present for it. Just pure taste, unfolding moment by moment. My Pleasure Eater had taken over my consciousness. It was orchestrating my every move, shaping my thoughts, and focusing my attention on the rich, comforting, and delightful experience of eating. It was a glorious meal. One that I still remember fondly.

That night, my Pleasure Eater gave me a glimpse of its gifts: how it can heighten awareness, amplify joy, and make eating feel like an art form. But what happens when the same force that makes a scallop feel transcendent can, under different conditions, drive me into mindless excess? What about when it urged me toward dessert despite feeling uncomfortably full? Or how can the same part of me that appreciates a Michelin-starred chef's subtle genius also crave artificial cheese powder?

The answers reveal something profound about how we perceive, navigate, and consume pleasure in a world designed to make pleasure endless.

Evolutionary Origins: Wired for Delight

The Pleasure Eater is an ancient impulse dressed in contemporary clothes. Our ancestors survived by pursuing calorie-dense foods—sweet fruits for quick energy, fatty meats for sustained fuel—while avoiding bitter compounds that often signaled toxins. This biological programming made perfect sense when high-calorie food was scarce.

Fast forward to today, and that same Pleasure Eater—evolved for scarcity—now navigates unprecedented abundance. What was once a vital survival tool has become both a blessing and a burden in our modern food landscape. Nowadays, we shop for eating experiences like we shop for clothes: seeking trendy restaurants, innovative dishes, and creative combinations to make us feel good. Food tourism, social media #foodporn, and celebrity chefs reflect a cultural preoccupation with taste as something to consume and flaunt.

With restaurants galore and takeout at the click of a button, our Pleasure Eaters inhabit a garden of earthly delights. I certainly wouldn't want to give up my freedom to eat Italian one night, Japanese the next, and Greek the following. Diversity is the spice to which my Pleasure Eater has become accustomed.

Yet this abundance of choice and cuisines challenges our temperance. Food 2.0 has weaponized pleasurable flavors, textures, and aromas, as discussed in previous chapters. Our inclinations have been emboldened from eating to overeating, from liking to wanting, and from enjoying to craving. The "flavor dust" and intoxicating aroma (think: Cinnabon) of Food 2.0 deliver dopamine spikes that pull our Pleasure Eaters to seek more. At the same time, bliss points kick our brain's opioid system into overdrive, producing a wave of soothing, feel-good sensations that are like a mini high. This powerful combo of dopamine and endogenous opioids can drive us to chase foods as if they're running away. Yet once secured in our hands, these delights are easy to overconsume without realizing it.

This poses the question: How do we reclaim our right to delight without losing sight of what might, by midnight, not feel right?

Recognizing the Voice of Your Pleasure Eater

Your Pleasure Eater has been operating your entire life, some-times whispering, sometimes shouting. Whenever you spit out food in disgust or think, *What flavor will taste the best?* this part is driving you. It's not checking nutritional labels; it wants what feels good, right now.

- *"Just one more bite—it's so yummy!"*
- *"Life is short. Let's eat cake."*
- *"What's going to taste best? I want the most flavorful option."*
- *"I deserve something delicious after the day I've had."*
- *"Have you tried that new restaurant? The food is so good."*
- *"Bad day? Chocolate. Good day? Chocolate."*

Unlike your Survival Eater, which eats for efficiency, your Pleasure Eater eats for experience. You'll know your Pleasure Eater is active when:

- You are preoccupied with memories of meals that you want to eat again.

- You continue eating despite feeling physically full because something tastes too good to stop.

- You feel disappointed when meals don't deliver the flavor you imagined.

- You find yourself planning your day around particular food experiences or thinking about eating at your favorite restaurants.

- You regularly override other concerns (health, budget, convenience) in pursuit of specific delicious foods.

- You find yourself longing for familiar comfort foods, especially during times of stress.

The Wisdom of Your Pleasure Eater

Despite its potential excesses, the Pleasure Eater carries profound wisdom that enriches your relationship with food. As activist adrienne maree brown notes, "Pleasure is a natural, safe, and liberated part of life."[1] At its best, our Pleasure Eater is our connection to this liberated part of life, and what a shame to deny ourselves this fundamental joy.

When we embrace and empower our Pleasure Eater, we also gain access to these gifts.

Enhancing mindfulness. In a world increasingly mediated through screens, the Pleasure Eater grounds us in direct sensory experience: the fundamental aliveness of taste, smell, and texture. When you savor each bite, you may find yourself eating less but enjoying your food more.

Elevating food into an experience. Cooking becomes creative, playful, and expressive. Your kitchen becomes your workshop, and every ingredient is a tool for the adventure. Eating out is like going to a movie—an experience that cannot be fully recreated at home, often due to the use of exotic ingredients, creative artistry, and careful presentation.

True enjoyment and satisfaction. When pleasure is allowed and appreciated, restriction loses its grip. A developed Pleasure Eater can distinguish between empty stimulation and genuine quality, letting the experience of pleasure fill you up as much as the calories.

The Shadow Side of the Pleasure Eater: When Pleasure Becomes Pain

The Pleasure Eater's shadow emerges when its natural drive for enjoyment becomes disconnected from true satisfaction. When pleasure is used as a coping mechanism, food stops being about joy and starts being about relief. A rough day at work? Ice cream. Feeling lonely? Chips. Stressed out? A cocktail and fries.

If food is your primary or only source of comfort, your Pleasure Eater will demand it more and more, expecting food to fix every emotional dip. This isn't wrong, but it can become a habit with significant physical and emotional costs. Like any single solution asked to solve multiple problems, food will eventually buckle under the weight of expectations it was never meant to carry.

If you've been taught to distrust pleasure, you may feel the urge to deny, delay, or micromanage every indulgence, creating imbalance. The result is a tumultuous relationship with your Pleasure Eater that swings between treating yourself and denying yourself. One day you're virtuously refusing the office birthday cake, the next you're standing in your kitchen at 10 PM eating ice cream straight from the container.

To help your Pleasure Eater find balance, you need to understand that it is vulnerable to the following pitfalls on the path to pleasure.

Hedonic adaptation. Like a song you once loved becoming something you barely notice, the first bite of cheese-dusted chips might be incredible, but by the tenth, your brain has adapted. Hedonic adaptation causes you to need more stimulation to get the same emotional impact. Your once-favorite foods may leave you unsatisfied if you eat them too often, leading you to eat more or crave bigger, bolder flavors.

Pleasure without presence. When pleasure isn't consciously registered, it stops being pleasure; it just becomes consumption. You may get a hint of that good feeling, but without mindfulness, it never lands.

Pleasure as escape: The Pleasure Eater can morph from a celebrator of life to an escape artist who uses food sensations to numb uncomfortable emotions. It says: *"I'm stressed, lonely, and bored. Let's eat."*

"Clean" vs "Dirty" Pleasure

All eating is emotional. The crucial distinction is whether we eat *with* emotions or *in reaction to* them. The former lends itself to "clean" pleasure that arises naturally. For instance, biting into a ripe peach, savoring it with slow bites, noticing the sweetness, the texture, and the juice. This clean pleasure is grounded in sensation and leaves you feeling satisfied. When the meal is over and the pleasure is gone, there is no mess for you to clean up.

"Dirty" pleasure, by contrast, often feels good at first, but masks something deeper, such as anger, loneliness, or grief. Dirty pleasure bypasses your conscious leadership.

Another way to think of dirty pleasure is pleasure without consent from all your Inner Eaters. You don't choose it. It chooses you. You grasp for it, fast and automatic, trying to outrun what you don't want to feel. It leaves behind restlessness, regret, or a stomach that's uncomfortably full.

Here's how that looked in my life: When the pressure of fatherhood or the stress of work pressed on my chest, I'd reach for the jar of seasoned nuts. One handful gave me instant relief. My Pleasure Eater knew the pattern: crunchy, oily, salty—followed by a moment where I didn't have to worry about a million things. It was temporary relief.

But the moment didn't last. One handful became three. Then five. Food 2.0 turbocharged the process by adding spices, yeast extract, sugar, and vinegar to light up every possible taste receptor in my mouth. Moreover, it sold me the family sized jar with twenty-eight servings, overriding any natural stopping point, allowing me to eat to my heart's content (or should I say, *discontent*). Soon enough, the jar was empty, my fingers were coated in addictive seasoning, and I still wasn't okay. My other Inner Eaters whispered: *"This isn't what we need."* But my Pleasure Eater had hijacked the system. It was running the show.

This isn't about demonizing emotional eating. Food *should* bring comfort. My Pleasure Eater developed these habits to protect me when life felt overwhelming. The challenge was that I had no say in the matter when I was lost in my Pleasure Eater's feeding frenzy. Over the years, I learned that I didn't need to immediately act on my Pleasure Eater's urges, or banish it from my life. I just needed to upgrade my relationship with it.

So, when seeking pleasure becomes compulsion, when you can't stop even as it stops serving you, that's your cue to ask: *What might be possible if I led my Pleasure Eater differently?*

Your Pleasure Eater's Personal History

Understanding your Pleasure Eater means examining your relationship with pleasure itself. For years I believed that I needed to "earn" food pleasure through restriction or exercise. I carefully calculated and doled out pleasure depending on how much work I put in. A decadent dinner meant restriction earlier in the day. A tasty treat would be inhaled in the corner of the kitchen as if hiding somehow made the act of eating less real. (Maybe no one would see me enjoying it; therefore, it didn't count.)

These behaviors were not accidental. Many were vestiges from my earlier eating disorder that left me completely pleasure-deprived. There were also numerous factors at play influencing the ways pleasure gets twisted with privilege, social conditioning, and self-worth. Western society has had a capricious attitude toward sensory gratification, which has been at different times disgraced, then glorified, shamed, then celebrated. This drama plays out inside many of us every time we decide how to satisfy our hunger.

To suss out your overall views about pleasure, take a moment to ask yourself:

- *Do I feel entitled to pleasure, or must I earn it?*
- *Is food joy something I receive with gratitude or guilt?*
- *Do I trust myself to experience pleasure without losing control?*
- *Do I limit how much enjoyment I allow myself?*
- *Have I ever used food as a substitute for other unmet pleasures in life?*

Unpacking your beliefs (and potential trauma or emotional baggage) around pleasure is vital to genuinely getting to know your Pleasure Eater. If you don't understand the ways you lean into pleasure or shy away from it, you'll never be able to lead your Pleasure Eater effectively.

I had to sort through a lot of internalized contradictory messages about pleasure to figure out why I felt restricted until I "earned it." If you don't resolve the underlying anxieties that drive your Pleasure Eater to indulgence and restriction, the cycle will inevitably repeat itself.

The American Pleasure Eater:
A Conflicted Appetite

The American relationship with food pleasure resembles a carnival funhouse mirror: distorted and confusing. Walk into a grocery store, and you'll see low-calorie, guilt-free ice cream sold in family-sized tubs. A fast-food commercial tells you to "treat yourself," but the culture around you says, "Don't get fat."

This quintessential American contradiction—where the Pleasure Eater is simultaneously glorified and shamed—is deliberately maintained by two powerful forces: the first, a food industry that romanticizes extreme indulgence and sells highly engineered flavors; and the second, a diet-fitness-beauty industry that promotes ageist, racist, and fatphobic body ideals. Both industries profit from keeping us in limbo, caught between desire and discipline, unsure whether to savor or suppress. These invisible scripts surround us, and they produce one thing: shame about our bodies, our food choices, and our right to enjoy food.

This shame lives within a complex web of cultural beliefs about:

Worthiness. The question of whether we deserve pleasure often underlies our relationship with self-worth. Food is love, and if you have internalized messages around your own worthiness (or lack thereof), it may complicate your ability to receive pleasure through food.

Morality. Some cultural and religious traditions frame pleasure, primarily physical, sensual pleasure, in moral terms. Indulgence is "sinful" or "decadent," while restraint is "virtuous" or "pure." Does eating to feel good violate a religious belief or make you less holy?

Control. For many, especially in achievement-oriented societies, controlled indulgence represents a victory over our brutish, uncivilized impulses. "Giving in" to pleasure signals weakness or failure to control these uncouth urges.

Class and status. Our Pleasure Eaters absorb messages about which food pleasures are sophisticated versus crass, proper versus improper. Think of the distinction between being a "foodie" versus a "junk food junkie." One is high-class. The other is derogatory and low-brow.

The result is that many people feel at war with their own Pleasure Eater. They either give in too much or deny themselves completely. Problems arise if your Pleasure Eater feels micromanaged and unable to express itself. When you overcontrol this part, it will respond like a teenager under curfew: It rebels, bargains for more, and flouts restrictions simply because it can. Given unexpected freedom—at buffets, parties, or when alone—it may take off running, leading to episodes of uninhibited consumption.

The truth is that pleasure was never supposed to be an all-or-nothing battle. In many other cultures, excessive gratification followed by self-shaming guilt isn't normal. The concept of "good" and "bad" foods may seem strange and foreign. In part, this is because many nations do not have the same saturation of Food 2.0 as we do in America. But more so, many other cultures support mindful enjoyment over mindless consumption. The French, for instance, enjoy rich foods while maintaining good health outcomes because they don't eat while distracted or shame pleasurable foods. The Japanese concept of *hara hachi bu* encourages eating until 80 percent full, recognizing that pleasure doesn't require over-the-top, Instagramable dishes that contain 3,500 calories and a stomach ache. These traditions remind us that pleasure need not be sinful or divorced from moderation. Yet, within mainstream American culture, it can feel impossible to navigate food pleasure without falling into excess.

The Imprint of Early Messages:
Steve's Story

Steve grew up in a household where pleasure was viewed with suspicion. "Dessert was for birthdays only," he recalls. "My mother would say, 'We don't eat those foods. They're not for us.' But then I'd go to friends' houses where dessert was normal, and eating was never 'bad' or 'too much.' I developed this split personality around food—publicly restricting, privately indulging in everything 'forbidden' whenever I had the chance."

For years, Steve oscillated between denial and excess. "I'd be 'good' for weeks, then find myself at 11 PM eating an entire package of cookies straight from the box, standing over the kitchen sink so no one would see the crumbs." This pattern continued until Steve recognized how deeply his mother's attitudes, shaped by her own cultural and economic background, had programmed his relationship with food pleasure.

Over time, Steve learned that the real solution wasn't more restriction or unlimited indulgence. He needed his Pleasure Eater to recognize and trust his adult reality. When he stopped making pleasure the enemy, he began the process of figuring out which foods actually brought him pleasure and which foods he could easily pass up. "Now, dessert isn't forbidden, but it's also not an all-or-nothing event. It's been a healing journey. I needed this part of me to believe I could enjoy good food without losing control. I had to release the shame and give it evidence that I'm a different guy than I was in the past. This has made all the difference."

The Developmental Age of Your Pleasure Eater

Steve's story demonstrates how our relationship with food pleasure carries the imprints of our earliest experiences and the cultural messages that shaped them. This raises two important questions: What internalized messages is your Pleasure Eater carrying? What developmental age is your Pleasure Eater operating from?

When people find themselves in the grips of their Pleasure Eater, they're often unconsciously searching for that uncomplicated joy they experienced as children. Often, the hankering for a special treat at the end of the day is your Pleasure Eater saying, *"Hey, don't forget about me!"* It aims to recreate a time when food didn't carry emotional baggage or when eating wasn't complicated by societal judgment or body image concerns—A time when food pleasure was clean, straightforward, and innocent.

Yet, as adults, we must navigate through layers of worthiness, appropriate indulgence, and deserving pleasure. In extreme cases, this creates a painful bipolar pattern where indulgence becomes secretive and shameful rather than an integrated part of a balanced life.

If you're feeling really out of balance with your eating—eating multiple pints of ice cream straight from the container and then wanting to throw up, hiding candy wrappers in secrecy, or sneaking midnight snacks out of fear of judgement—it may be a sign of something deeper and time to seek professional support. Eating disorders are serious mental health conditions that require treatment. You are not to blame. Help is available, and recovery is possible

Even if your Pleasure Eater feels balanced, it helps to examine where your attitudes toward food came from. You can then choose which beliefs still serve you and which deserve reconsideration. This frees your Pleasure Eater to enjoy food fully, unlocking childlike joy while letting go of outdated or unhelpful ideas.

The Protective Palette:
Understanding Picky Eating

Your Pleasure Eater doesn't just seek delight; it also defends against disgust. The same instinct that craves your favorite flavors can just as fiercely reject unfamiliar ones. A child refusing mushy peas and an adult cringing at a foreign dish are acting from the same impulse: to protect pleasure and avoid discomfort.

Picky eating is a Pleasure Eater's defense mechanism. It says, *"I know what I like, and this isn't it."* Sometimes, the aversion is about smell or texture. Other times, it's tied to a memory: A dish once forced on you might never feel like *your* choice. (The casserole your aunt insisted you eat might be why you still avoid it.) For some, picky eating is about control. Saying *no* to certain foods reinforces a sense of agency, a clarity many lose to social pressure or nutrition trends.

Pickiness and preference go hand in hand, but when your Pleasure Eater becomes too rigid, your food world shrinks. Eating becomes tinged with fear of the unknown. The list of unappealing flavors balloons, and your palate becomes inured to a few foods that you deem tolerable.

The pursuit of pleasure and the avoidance of pain both need to be honored and tempered wisely. The goal isn't forcing yourself to like everything, but you must also learn when your aversions are real and when they're reflexes built on untested or outdated assumptions.

Alex, a self-described meat-and-potatoes guy, explains: "I know there's amazing food from all these different countries, but when I try something unfamiliar, all I taste is 'wrong.' It's not even that it's bad; It just doesn't work for me. I avoid it. It's like 'why bother?'"

To lead your Pleasure Eater wisely, you must balance comfort with curiosity. Some dislikes are valid, especially if you're among a small population of "supertasters" who have an outsized perception of flavor. Still, other disliked foods may be old memories that are waiting for a second chance, being prepared the right way, at the right time.

Leading Your Pleasure Eater Wisely

Developing a mature relationship with your Pleasure Eater means guiding it toward its highest expression. The CARE model offers a compassionate roadmap for working with your Pleasure Eater without shame, willpower games, or swinging between indulgence and restriction.

Imagine coming home after a stressful day at work. It's 9:30 PM. You've already eaten dinner. You're not hungry. But the kids are asleep, and you've been thinking about the chocolate in your pantry for the last hour. Before you know it, you're standing in the kitchen with an empty wrapper, barely remembering the experience of eating it.

You're not a failure for wanting it. You're human. And your Pleasure Eater is doing what it's designed to do: seek joy, comfort, and release from the weight of the day. The question isn't whether this part of you is good or bad. The question is: Is this a conscious choice or an ingrained habit?

CURIOSITY:
GET TO KNOW YOUR DESIRE

Become your Pleasure Eater's witness by creating a space between the desire to eat and the action itself. This space shifts you from being *inside* the craving to *observing* it from the seat of awareness. It's not about suppressing the desire. It's about seeing what it's trying to say. Often, your Pleasure Eater is trying to soothe your tired, weary soul using the only tool it knows: mouth sensation.

ONE PRACTICE:
THE PAUSE AND THREE QUESTIONS

Before you reach for a piece of food—especially at night, during emotional moments, or out of habit, set a timer for one minute. Place your hand over your heart, and during that time, ask yourself the following three questions.

- *Where is this desire coming from—stomach, emotion, or memory?*
- *What need is my Pleasure Eater trying to meet?*
- *Does food meet this need? If not, what else is possible?*

APPRECIATION:
CARING FOR THE PART THAT CARES FOR YOU

Most people either obey the Pleasure Eater blindly or shame it for showing up. Eating 2.0 offers a third way: Appreciate its intent. It wants life to be joyful, exuberant, and fun—I don't think anyone would argue against that.

ONE PRACTICE:
THE DAILY ACKNOWLEDGMENT

Step into your role of conscious leader and talk directly to your Pleasure Eater. When you notice your Pleasure Eater emerging (through cravings, comfort food impulses, or the urge to indulge), you can say something like: *Thank you for bringing me comfort. Thank you for reminding me that "adulting" doesn't mean sacrificing fun and flavor. I see you. I feel you. You've helped me through a lot.*

Then, take a full breath. Practice this acknowledgment at least once daily for two weeks. See if your Pleasure Eater becomes less demanding and more willing to collaborate.

RESPONSIBILITY:
OWNING YOUR PLEASURE

The mature Pleasure Eater understands that food choices have consequences, not just in the moment but over time. Taking responsibility doesn't mean abandoning special treats; it means conscious ownership of your pleasure and its impact on your entire Inner Eater family.

ONE PRACTICE:
THE PLEASURE-CONSEQUENCE JOURNAL

To assess the value of your three most cherished indulgences, create a simple two-columned entry in a journal or on a notepad.

In the first column, write specifically what you love about this food or eating experience.

In the second column, honestly document how you feel one hour and one day after consuming it.

After seven days of this practice, create a third column where you design your personal "sweet spot" —the amount of the food and the context to eat it in that maximizes (clean) pleasure while minimizing unwanted (dirty) consequences. This is not about earning it or giving yourself permission to eat, but about ensuring your pleasure remains truly pleasurable.

EXPLORATION:
LET'S PLAY WITH THE EDGES.

Your Pleasure Eater is constantly guiding you towards delight. Not every night will be the same. Some nights, ice cream is exactly what you need. Other nights, it's a decoy. The only way to know the difference is to experiment consciously and build feedback loops around your choices.

ONE PRACTICE:
THE 10 PERCENT WEEKLY EXPERIMENT

Choose one pleasurable food habit to modify using the 10 percent rule. This might be:
- Reduce the portion size by 10 percent.
- Slow the pace of your eating by 10 percent.
- Change the setting by 10 percent.
- Savor the first and last 10 percent of what you eat.

- Substitute 10 percent of a food with a new alternative.
- Delay your indulgence by ten minutes.

The more you explore, the more refined your palate and your self-trust will become. It's helpful to treat your Pleasure Eater like a creative partner. The objective of exploration is to discover what rituals, flavors, and boundaries bring you clean pleasure. This is the heart of Eating 2.0: adaptive, embodied, feedback-driven wisdom.

After seven days, evaluate: Was this 10 percent shift beneficial? Should you continue, adjust, or try a different experiment next week?

Remember, your Pleasure Eater isn't just here for chocolate or chips. It's here to help you remember that joy, when guided wisely, is not a distraction from the path. It *is* the path.

Looking Ahead:
From Personal Pleasure to Social Connection

At its core, your Pleasure Eater constantly navigates between seeking joy and avoiding discomfort, chasing flavors, textures, and experiences that feel good while steering clear of anything that might bring disgust or disappointment.

Taking CARE of your Pleasure Eater means becoming the leader who knows how to savor, pause, and choose good flavors from a place of alignment. But here's the plot twist: Your Pleasure Eater has more company than your Survival Eater.

Just when you think you've matured your relationship with pleasure, the Social Eater enters the picture, adding a whole new element to your eating. Now, pleasure isn't just about what tastes good; it's also about who you're eating with, what's expected of you, and how you fit in. Eating a burger alone at home is one thing. Eating a burger at a backyard cookout, where passing on it feels like rejecting friendship itself? That's another.

The people around you—family, friends, coworkers, even strangers at dinner parties—become invisible hands shaping your food choices. Sometimes, they encourage indulgence ("Come on, one more bite, you have to try this!"). Other times, they reinforce restriction ("Wow, you're really going to eat that?"). We will explore all of this and more in the next chapter, so turn the page and join me, because eating isn't just about hunger, it's about connection.

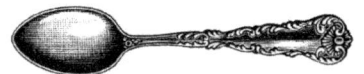

SEVEN

YOUR SOCIAL EATER
THE BELONGING SEEKER WHO FEARS BEING LEFT OUT

"Food is maybe the only universal thing that really has the power to bring everyone together. No matter what culture, everywhere around the world, people eat together."

GUY FIERI

I was already sweating when I sat down. Not from the heat, but from the tension of being an outsider at a dinner I didn't understand. I was a young American in Penang, Malaysia, invited to a friend's family meal. He'd told me only this: "My mom's an amazing cook. Trust us."

"*Us*," I thought to myself. *Who else is going to be there?*

The dining room had no table, just an ornate cloth spread across the floor. I was placed to the right of the host, the seat of honor, though I didn't know this at the time. Around me, people settled into prescribed positions: Men sat cross-legged; women tucked their legs to the side like mermaids. I, meanwhile, dropped into a squat like I was waiting for a campfire story.

There were no plates. Just banana leaves. No forks or knives. Just hands.

Food was spooned onto my leaf: steaming rice, tangy pickles, lentils, papadum. It smelled incredible. But as I watched the others deftly ball their rice and scoop soupy curries into their mouths, I panicked. I mimicked their motions, fumbling to form a bite. Then, mid-mouthful, my friend leaned over and whispered, "Right hand only. The left is . . . *uh* . . . unclean."

But I'm left-handed.

Each bite became a feat of awkward contortion. I dropped food. I dribbled. I tried to smile, pretending I wasn't embarrassed. But I kept eating.

I didn't want to offend anyone or be the foreigner who couldn't handle the spice. I felt compelled to finish the food that was served, not because I was hungry, but because everyone else was still eating.

That night, my Social Eater was in charge. This part of me wasn't thinking about nutrients or flavors. It was thinking about *belonging*. It wanted to eat its way to acceptance, in this case, by honoring the invisible rules of a food culture I didn't yet understand.

What this part knew so well is that when someone feeds you, they're offering more than food—they're offering connection.

As Mexican-American farmworker César Chávez once said, "If you really want to make a friend, go to someone's house and eat with him . . . The people who give you their food give you their heart."[1]

My friend's family had offered their heart, and this meal wasn't about taste. It was about trust. Trusting *us*.

Yet I hesitated: Could I trust them? Could I trust their food? Even deeper: Could I trust myself to eat in a way that met my needs and *their expectations?*

Evolutionary Origins: Wired for Connection

Long before restaurants, community cookouts, or supper clubs, humans were social eaters. Our survival depended not just on what we ate *but who we ate with.*

In mammals, feeding is fused with bonding, attachment, and physical intimacy. Nursing doesn't just deliver nutrients; it delivers safety. As an infant, eating is about gazing into your caregiver's eyes, feeling their attunement to your hunger and fullness, and experiencing the profound security of being nourished by another human being.

These early experiences create what attachment theorists call *internal working models* that shape your lifelong relationship with food as a vehicle for connection. A responsive caregiver who respected your hunger and fullness cues likely fostered a secure attachment in you to both food and relationships. When you could trust that your caregiver would tend to your hunger, your body released oxytocin, a hormone that promotes bonding, relaxation, and connection. In the language of neurotransmitters, if dopamine is the primary driver of your Pleasure Eater, oxytocin is the primary driver of your Social Eater, increasing social trust and allowing you to settle into your meals with others.

Beyond mother-child bonding, eating and connection have been inseparable since prehistoric times. Primitive humans survived not because they were the fastest or strongest species but because they collaborated to overcome hunger. Our ancestors shared kills, foraged in groups, cooked around fires, and organized themselves around rituals of provision and protection.[2] Eating together meant staying alive. To be excluded from the meal was a death sentence.

This ancient wiring still lives inside you. In fact, eating together is one of the most potent forms of nervous system synchrony. When you feel safe enough to eat together, you can relax your vigilance against predators and threats. There's a bidirectional relationship: Sharing food creates a sense of safety, and feeling safe allows you to truly share food.

That's why family dinners matter. It's why first dates happen over meals. It's why cultures have developed rich, elaborate rituals around how food is prepared, served, and eaten. Research from the World Happiness Report found that knowing how many meals someone shares with others reveals more about their well-being than knowing their income. Yes, shared meals predict happiness better than wealth.[3]

Your Social Eater understands this profound truth—that breaking bread together nourishes not just your body, but also your emotional resilience and sense of connectedness. If your Survival Eater is concerned about the nutrients on your plate, then your Social Eater is paying attention to the relationships encoded in every bite.

But here's where things get complicated in the modern world. You might be an Italian eating Japanese food in Brazil while FaceTiming someone in New York. Or your dining partner is keto, you're plant-based, and the person next to you is fasting till noon. Who sets the rules when there's no coherent food culture? What tribe do you belong to if you eat meat one day but not the next? And what happens when someone else's appetite overrides your hunger?

A groundbreaking study in the journal *Appetite* definitively answered that last question. Researchers seated people who hadn't eaten for twenty-four hours next to either "big eaters" or "small eaters." After offering unlimited food, the results were startling: Hunger didn't drive behavior, social context did. Even ravenously hungry participants ate little when seated beside someone who ate sparingly. Conversely, people who sat next to a "big eater" consumed a lot more food, regardless of how hungry they were.[4] The takeaway is that your tablemate's appetite, not your empty stomach, might dictate how much you eat.

This finding echoes the groundbreaking work of Nicholas Christakis and James Fowler, who showed that health behaviors and the weight changes that emanate from them can spread through social networks almost like a virus. Their studies found that when a friend becomes obese, an individual's own likelihood of becoming obese increases by approximately 57 percent, even if you live miles apart.[5] In other words, the choices of people around you ripple outward, shaping your own appetite, expectations, and sense of what's "normal."

This is what makes the Social Eater such a stealthy character. It's remarkably adaptive, operating under our awareness to blend into our social context, but in a globalized, fractured, Food 2.0 world, it can lose track of what's appropriate or necessary. It may guide you to seek belonging with fans of the next fad diet, viral food trends, or Instagram influencers. This powerful social pull can quietly override your actual needs, twist your choices, and leave you socially fitting but physically off.

Recognizing the Voice of Your Social Eater

Learning to spot your Social Eater in action will help you finally understand the invisible force that's been guiding your food choices at shared meals and social outings. It will save you from meals where you walk away thinking, *Why did I keep eating? Did I even want that last bite?*

Start by watching the people at your table. You may begin to notice an invisible rhythm, a social dance you didn't know you were doing.

Here are some common behaviors and internal dialogues to notice at your next communal meal.

Behavior. You eat because others are eating—even if you're not hungry.
Inner voice. *I'll just have a few more bites since others are still eating.*

Behavior. You feel uneasy saying no to food someone offers.
Inner voice. *I can't be the only one not eating, drinking, or having seconds. They'll think I'm rude if I don't try it. I don't want to be difficult by mentioning my dietary needs.*

Behavior. You match your pace, portions, or choices to those around you.
Inner voice. *Follow their lead. Are they going back for more? Do they still have food on their plate?*

Behavior. You eat foods you wouldn't choose alone to foster connection.
Inner voice. *Let's get share plates—Make everyone feel included.*

Behavior. You use food preparation as a primary way to express love and care, or as a means to connect with your cultural or family identity.
Internal dialogue. *I made this from scratch, the old way. It's Grandma's recipe. I hope everyone appreciates the effort.*

Your Social Eater often shows up strongest when the social script is thick with meaning and the stakes of belonging are high, such as when:

- Eating with large groups (such as at family dinners, shared meals, reunions).

- In unfamiliar environments or event spaces (such as in offices, cafeterias, stadiums, wedding venues, or school auditoriums).

- Sampling foreign or "exotic" cuisines (while traveling, at ethnic restaurants, or as a guest in someone's home— like my experience in a friend's house in Malaysia).

- Eating in public, especially in places not designed for meals (such as in planes, churches, trains, and courtrooms).

- Participating in ritual or ceremonial meals (like Shabbat, Iftar, Thanksgiving, Passover Seder, and Easter dinner).

At holiday tables and ceremonial meals, food becomes symbolic. It carries memory, meaning, and more often than not, a silent pressure to conform. Declining the offering might feel like declining the love behind it. To eat differently might feel like stepping outside the circle of care. In those moments—maybe even without realizing it—a part of you adapts to fit in.

The Wisdom of Your Social Eater

At its best, your Social Eater is a diplomat, fluent in the nuances of togetherness. It understands that food is a language of belonging, a tangible expression of care, and a bridge between differences.

When operating from these gifts, your Social Eater:

Creates meaningful rituals. The Thanksgiving turkey prepared using the family recipe; the birthday cake, which must be chocolate with buttercream frosting because that's how Mom demands it; and the family dinners that provide rhythm to life. My family has been doing Taco Tuesdays for years, and this weekly ritual creates familiarity in a changing world. It's an al pastor occasion that my wife and son have grown to love.

Fosters inclusion and acceptance. Your Social Eater recognizes food as a universal language that can transcend barriers. The careful consideration of a guest's dietary restrictions, the offering of food to a new neighbor, the potluck where everyone contributes something meaningful—these acts say "you belong here" in a way that words alone cannot.

Builds community resilience. Throughout human history, communities that shared food developed stronger social networks that helped them weather hardships. From neighborhood cookouts to meal trains for new parents or bereaved families, your Social Eater recognizes food as a concrete way to strengthen the social fabric. The more meals you share with someone, the closer you feel—oxytocin increases bonding.

Enhances enjoyment through shared experience. Your Social Eater intuitively knows that food is more flavorful and satisfying when shared. Research has shown that people who eat more meals with others tend to be more satisfied with their lives and are more likely to express positive emotions—regardless of culture, age, or demographics. To put it another way, if you want to get the most out of your money, don't dine at fancy Michelin-star restaurants alone.

Expands your culinary horizons. Your Social Eater's desire for connection often leads to culinary adventures you might otherwise avoid. Friends, partners, or colleagues from different backgrounds can expose you to new foods or new restaurants that expand your repertoire of tasty and enjoyable dishes.

The Shadow Side of Social Eating: Vulnerabilities and Shortcomings

When your Social Eater loses its rightful place in your Inner Eater family, it swings to extremes: excessive accommodation or rigid rebellion, both sacrificing authenticity for the illusion of safety or independence.

THE APPEASER

This version of your Social Eater is a people-pleaser. It prioritizes harmony over honesty—mimicking what others eat, when they eat, and how much they eat. This part is preoccupied with blending in to stay safe inside the group.

Take Will. It was his first team dinner at a new job, a chance to make a good impression. When his boss ordered a local IPA, Will nodded to indicate "I'll have the same." He wasn't in the mood for beer, but it wasn't about preference; it was about signaling *I belong*.

When appetizers came around, Will took the bread and calamari. Turning them down felt risky, even rude.

By the time his honey-glazed pork chop arrived—a dish his boss had recommended—Will had already overridden every internal cue to stop eating foods that disagreed with his system. He left the table uncomfortably full and a little disconnected from himself. But his Social Eater whispered: *"Great meal. Positive impressions. Good job."*

The Appeaser says *yes* when you mean *maybe*. It nods, smiles, and chews, even when your body says *no*.

Its fear? Saying *what you really want* might disrupt the connection. Your preferences might be *too much, too inconvenient,* or *too different.*

You'll often find the Appeaser:

- Eating past fullness to match others' appetite.
- Accepting food that doesn't sit well or align with your values.
- Minimizing dietary needs to avoid "making it a thing."
- Using food to soften tension or sidestep conflict.
- Confusing flexibility with self-erasure.

THE CONTRARIAN

At the other end of the spectrum from the Appeaser, your Social Eater can rebel, rejecting food norms out of protest. It turns meals into stages for autonomy and identity performance. This part doesn't just eat differently; it makes sure everyone sees you doing it.

Take Anna as an example. She grew up in a Southern family where meals meant strict tradition and clean plates. Meat was a mainstay, and veggies were scarce. However, a few of Anna's friends at school became vegetarians, and she chose to be with her peers over her family.

By doing so, she refused the food everyone in her family loved. By adolescence, family meals became a battleground, especially with her mom, who did most of the cooking.

"I wasn't just skipping dishes," she recalls. "I was pushing back. Making a point. Proving I didn't belong to their world anymore."

By the time she was sixteen, she exaggerated her dislikes and chose the one diet that would guarantee a clash at the table. She became vegan. In hindsight, Anna admits: "I was still letting their expectations dictate my choices—just in reverse."

As an adult, Anna's Social Eater was still a rebellious teenager looking for belonging outside her family of origin. She hated sharing food and always wanted something different from the group. Moreover, she wasn't shy about letting you know. Anna had become a real pain in the ass around shared meals; she had developed a grandiose contrarian Social Eater.

You'll often find the Contrarian:

- Making food choices primarily to annoy or differentiate from others.
- Forfeiting social connection for control.
- Missing chances for shared joy.
- Judging others' choices to feel superior.
- Wielding food rules like armor to protect deeper insecurities.

What's the fear driving this zealous behavior? *If I compromise, I'll be absorbed and erased by the group. If I eat what you eat, I can't be better than you.*

The extremes of both the Appeaser and the Contrarian stem from attachment wounds related to approval and abandonment. Deep inside the shadow of this Social Eater lies programming that feels ashamed for taking up space or lacks trust in others. Updating this code means learning that authentic connection requires bringing your whole self—including your unique relationship with food—to the table, even if that looks different from the group.

Your Social Eater's Personal History

My wife and I often joke that there are two kinds of people in the world: those who share dishes and those who don't.

We're firmly in the sharing camp. When we go out to eat, we split everything—tasting, trading, experimenting. It's playful. We like to collaborate while dining out, sometimes choosing a dish neither of us would've ordered on our own.

Over the years, we've become skilled at balancing each other's preferences. You could say our Social Eaters have become highly attuned and synchronized—good teammates. Occasionally, we push each other past our comfort zones; other times, we return to familiar favorites. The shared meal becomes a dance: an eating metaphor for cocreative partnership.

But it wasn't always that way for me.

I grew up in a "everyone gets their own plate" kind of household. My mom, worn out from catering to picky preferences, used to sigh and say, "This is not a restaurant. I'm not cooking four different meals." Yet there was rarely one dish that satisfied everyone. My dad was rigid. My brother, stubborn. I was somewhere in between, but as my eating disorder became more severe, I stopped expressing any preference at all because I would barely eat. I convinced myself I was easygoing, but I was actually signaling: "My needs don't matter. You choose." That was a mask—a strategy my Social Eater developed to minimize conflict, avoid disappointment, and keep the peace in our household.

The unintended cost? My Social Eater gradually pushed my Pleasure Eater into the shadows. I stopped knowing what I really wanted. Expressing preferences felt risky. Saying "I'd actually rather have . . ." made me feel selfish, or worse, ungrateful. Even among friends, I'd defer when it came time to pick a restaurant or order a meal.

Eventually, it felt easier just to eat alone or not eat at all.

Years later, I learned that advocating for my preferences didn't make me difficult; it made me whole. Healing included letting go of old fears, such as fear of rocking the boat, being judged, or not seeming "manly" enough if I ordered a salad. If I could go back in time, I would tell my younger self that *his needs did matter*, his hunger was valid, and his worth had nothing to do with how he ate. The beautiful part is that I don't have to time travel to practice this. The residues of my teenage self still live inside my Social Eater. Now, when I notice patterns of overaccommodating or erasing my food preferences, I can meet this part with love and kindness, giving it what it never got as a kid. I can help it break free from cultural scripts that mistakenly tether value to how you eat and how you look. When I unburden it from unrealistic expectations it took on as a youngster, I help it return to its rightful place within my Inner Eater family.

I share this story because your Social Eater has a personal history, too. It may have lots of baggage from growing up with cultural or family dynamics that glorified one way of eating and shamed others. Understanding your social eating history is the first step to upgrading it.

FIVE FACETS OF YOUR SOCIAL EATER'S PATTERNS

Your Social Eater has been shaped by every meal with your family, every school lunch, every awkward first date, and every group meal where you scanned the room to figure out what was acceptable. Unpacking these experiences is essential to understanding why your Social Eater behaves as it does.

Here are five important factors to consider.

Your family's food culture: the dynamics, roles, and unspoken rules that governed your childhood table. Whether meals were formal or casual, silent or chatty, rushed or leisurely, combat zones or peace treaties, they all created your baseline expectations for how food and relationships intertwine.

Cultural expectations: messages about what people of your gender, race, class, or heritage were "supposed" to eat or enjoy. For many women, their Social Eater becomes entangled with caregiving expectations: the pressure to prioritize others' preferences, to derive satisfaction from providing food rather than consuming, and to demonstrate restraint around "indulgent" foods. For men, social eating often involves performances of masculinity, ordering the largest dish, or one-upping the other guy by eating and drinking more.

Body-related pressures: experiences of being judged, praised, or shamed based on your eating in relation to your appearance. Your Social Eater exists in dialogue with ever-shifting cultural ideals about which bodies deserve inclusion. These messages vary dramatically across cultures, generations, and communities, but they universally impact how freely people can engage with food in social settings.

Your relationship with food access: whether meals represented abundance or scarcity, choice or necessity. Your Social Eater's development has been profoundly influenced by the socio-economic context of your upbringing. Food availability shapes not only what you eat, but also whether meals feel precious, sacred, or scattered.

Heritage and belonging: how traditional foods connect you to (or distance you from) your cultural identity. For many, particularly those from first-generation immigrant families or minority cultures, food traditions become vital anchors of identity. Your Social Eater may look to particular foods and ways of eating that signal belonging in environments that may otherwise feel alienating.

Once you understand your Social Eater's history, you'll stop taking its reactions personally and start seeing them as information, data you can use to make more conscious choices at your very next meal. It can be useful to inquire: *What old stories might be driving my Social Eater's choices today?*

The One Person You Eat With the Most

Think about the one person you eat with the most: Your partner, your spouse, your roommate, your coworker, or your best friend. Their eating habits shape yours, often more than you realize.

- Do they eat late? You might shift your schedule.
- Do they like everything spicy? You build a tolerance.
- Do they prefer cooking from scratch or ordering in? You adapt.
- Do they clean their plate religiously? You feel guilty leaving food behind.
- Do they eat quickly? You speed up. Slowly? You linger longer.
- Do they eat in front of a screen? You pull out your phone.

Over time, these micro-adjustments mold your experience of eating. Your Social Eater is constantly navigating the tricky terrain of long-term relationships. Every meal it needs to decide when to flex, when to fold, when to speak up, and when to remain silent.

When You're the One Who Manages Meals: Parenting and Family

Your Social Eater transforms when tiny humans enter the picture. Suddenly, you're not just eating for yourself, you're feeding others, crafting their relationship with food while quietly reshaping your own.

Many parents (I know from first-hand experience) discover that their eating habits dramatically shift when children arrive. For example:

- You find yourself finishing the crumbs, crusts, half-eaten pieces, and abandoned snacks.

- You eat standing up in stolen moments of divided attention rather than seated at the table.

- Your meal choices narrow to what the "tiny tyrants" will accept.

- You save the "good stuff" for them, taking the burned piece, gristly section, or smaller portion for yourself.

- Your pace accelerates; eating quickly becomes a survival skill when parenting demands your attention.

When you're always in provider mode, your Social Eater may suppress your Pleasure Eater or Strategic Eater to make sure everyone else is fed. This creates inner turmoil that eventually bubbles out in all sorts of inconvenient ways. Your Strategic Eater might restrict your kids access to sugar or treats to "model healthy eating." Your Pleasure Eater might overindulge after bedtime when the pressure lifts. Your Social Eater may even cook separate meals for everyone to avoid battles. (This was my mom bemoaning the labor of feeding four different palates at dinner time.)

For many parents, meals become about control, compliance, or convenience rather than connection. Internally, your Inner Eaters are scrambling for scraps and arguing over who gets say in the meal.

The irony? You're trying to give your kids a healthy, joyful relationship with food while sacrificing your own.

Here is the deeper issue to pay attention to: Your kids are developing their own Social Eaters. If you tie eating to receiving attention, being "good," or gaining approval, your kids will internalize these messages. Understanding this is key because it quietly shapes how you feed your family, creating ripples that extend for generations. It is your responsibility to break the cycle of unconsciously passing on unspoken expectations of love and worth wrapped in food.

This doesn't mean abandoning all rules or boundaries at the table. (For example, we expect our son not to throw food, but we don't expect him to clean his plate.) It does mean consciously choosing which food rules, expectations, or traditions to keep and which to gently release. You must help your children not conflate your parental instruction, "This eating behavior is unacceptable," with the message, "You are unlovable because you eat this way." The deeper question is whether you're ready to give yourself the love you never got around eating so you can give it to your family.

Leading Your Social Eater Wisely

Imagine this common scenario: It's Sunday afternoon, and you're heading to your buddy's place to watch the game. You know the drill—chips, beer, wings, loaded nachos, and pizza will be spread across the table. The guys will be grabbing handfuls of snacks between plays, cracking open another beer during commercials, and nobody will be paying attention to how much they're eating.

181

Here's the game changer: You don't have to choose between conscious leadership and social connection. The CARE approach will help you feel genuinely satisfied, both physically and socially, at your next group meal by skillfully acknowledging and managing tensions rather than pretending they don't exist.

CURIOSITY:
SCOUT THE TERRITORY

Before heading to the gathering, take a moment to ask yourself: *What happens to my eating during these Sunday games? What social dynamics influence me the most here? Do I let my Social Eater take over? If so, does it become an "appeaser" or "contrarian"?*

ONE PRACTICE:
MATCHING AND MIRRORING

At your next social eating gathering, choose one person to subtly observe throughout the event. Notice when they eat, drink, pause, or reach for seconds. Then, notice if you follow similar patterns. Do you match your friends drink for drink and bite for bite? You don't need to change or fix anything; Just notice this part of you in operation. The moment you start observing instead of just reacting, you reclaim your power to act differently if you choose.

APPRECIATION:
VALUE THE TEAM SPIRIT

Your Social Eater isn't fumbling because you want connection. This part of you understands that sharing food and drink while cheering for your favorite team creates bonds that transcend the final score. This is especially true in a busy world where slowing down to spend time with friends has become increasingly rare. Lean into that sense of belonging and amplify it.

ONE PRACTICE:
CHAMPION CAMARADERIE

Identify what these gatherings bring to your life: A chance to maintain long-standing friendships? To catch-up? To reminisce? To gossip? To laugh? To vent? To cheer?

Also, identify what these gatherings give you emotionally, a sense of: Camaraderie? Continuity? Comfort? Relief? Validation? Safety?

Appreciate your Social Eater for trying to secure these feelings, and let it know: "I see your desire to get on well with others. Thank you." Honoring your Social Eater's positive intentions reduces internal conflict and self-criticism.

RESPONSIBILITY:
CALL YOUR OWN PLAYS

Taking responsibility means being the quarterback of your eating decisions rather than just following the team's momentum. You can fully participate in the camaraderie while still honoring your body's signals. It just takes practice in setting clear and respectful boundaries.

ONE PRACTICE:
SET APPROPRIATE BOUNDARIES

Before your next social gathering, decide on one clear boundary you'll maintain, and prepare a simple, confident response for when it's tested. Write it down and practice saying it aloud in a casual, matter-of-fact tone.

For example, you might decide to limit yourself to two drinks, enough to participate in the ritual but not so many that you'll feel terrible Monday morning. Internally, validate your Social Eater, letting it know its presence is appreciated and wanted at the party—you weren't invited over by accident.

Then, reassure your Social Eater that diverging from the group will not threaten your friendship. If people do push back, give you grief, or make it hard to honor your limits, that's your cue to hold strong or remove yourself from the situation. You are your own person. You're allowed to have your own opinions. No one else has to wake up in your body; therefore, no one else should have sway over what you put in it.

When it's time to reinforce a boundary, you step into your position at the head of the table and lead with calm confidence. In the case of being offered a third drink, say, "I'm good for now, thanks." No drama. Just clarity. Your Social Eater knows it's been heard. Rapport has been established, and it feels safe enough to say "No, thank you."

It is important to remember that you cannot control other people's responses to your boundary. If they don't react well, that is their emotional work to do, not yours. You may feel uncomfortable (and some people tend to be very pushy around food), but you should not let guilt get in the way of doing what's right for you.

EXPLORATION:
CREATE A NEW PLAYBOOK

Exploring means inventing new rituals of eating together, such as transforming peer pressure into creative possibility, wherein your Social Eater feels included and your Survival, Pleasure, and Strategic Eaters walk away satisfied, too.

ONE PRACTICE:
CONSCIOUSLY CONTRIBUTE TO THE MEAL

Choose one proactive contribution you can make to a shared meal, ideally something that strengthens connection *and* works for all your Inner Eaters.

In the football party example, if you know there will be chips and guacamole, instead of buying store-bought guacamole, you could get everyone involved in making your own. Bring avocados, limes, onions, and jalapenos to create a shared cooking and eating experience that checks off all the boxes: game-day bites, socializing with friends, and feeling good afterward.

Your Survival Eater might initially balk at the idea of making guac. *"Why go through all the trouble? Just buy the ready-to-eat stuff!"* But your Pleasure Eater, Social Eater, and Strategic Eater might prefer preparing food together with friends.

With all of this, the goal isn't magical alignment of your needs with everyone else's—you might still eat wings you don't particularly enjoy or feel pressured to have another beer. You might not follow your boundary or feel safe enough to say "no." That's okay. Remember, Eating 2.0 is about presence over perfection. Don't get bogged down in the minutia of a single eating experience.

What's more important than chips and guac is growing your capacity to lead your Social Eater wisely, with compassion rather than coercion. Stop holding yourself to unrealistic standards or expectations. You *want* to feel the tension between peer pressure and personal preference. This means you're doing the work of evolving, rewriting outdated scripts, and gathering evidence that belonging doesn't require self-abandonment.

Your Social Eater in the Food 2.0 World

Your Social Eater is working overtime because our Food 2.0 world has scrambled all its familiar signals.

Nowadays, you may gather around the table, but the table is likely to be in a chain restaurant, devoid of history. The meal might resemble a feast that your family cooked, but it lacks the depth of flavor or meaning from food that was prepared together, close to the land.

Even at home, the ritual of eating together has changed. Dinner might be microwaved leftovers, eaten side by side while scrolling your phone. The appearance of togetherness remains, but its depth is diluted. Your Social Eater shows up, eager to connect, but instead of rich cultural rhythms and cocreated meaning, it finds mindless bites.

This is the sleight of hand of Food 2.0: It preserves the *form* of social eating while hollowing out its *function*. The structure remains, but the relational nourishment is missing. Food choices and accompaniments that once signified cultural belonging—the chopsticks, rodízio, thali plates, banchan, bamboo steamers, and so forth—now function as consumer preferences. We consume the world's cuisines as entertainment rather than embodied heritage.

The wealth of options that seem to promise connection ("Do you want to try that new Indian takeout spot or go back to the Italian restaurant?") often leaves us eating globally while thinking individually. Just as our Pleasure Eater gets lured into eating more but enjoying it less, our Social Eater may yearn to eat together but feel increasingly disconnected.

Looking Ahead:
From Social Connection to Personal Achievement

As you get to know your Social Eater, you can notice when it's active and what it's seeking: tribe, trust, safety. Instead of blindly following its cues or exiling this part of you, you integrate it. You become the one who sets the tone, chooses the table, and creates new rituals that feed both body and spirit.

Something magical happens when you consciously lead in this manner. You can enjoy a birthday cake that connects you to your friends while honoring your survival needs and pleasure preferences. You can participate in boxed office lunches, linking fuel and fellowship without abandoning your dietary needs. You can explore new cuisines without losing your sense of self and the social customs you hold dear. This is the conscious leadership your Social Eater has been waiting for, and it prepares you for what comes next: your Strategic Eater.

If your Social Eater roots you in the collective moment, your Strategic Eater points toward the horizon. It's the part of you that asks, *"Who am I becoming through the way I eat?"* When you engage this next member of your Inner Eater family, meals transcend social connection, survival, and pleasure—they become a pathway toward your highest health and deepest values.

EIGHT

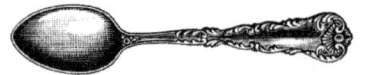

YOUR STRATEGIC EATER
THE AMBITIOUS PLANNER WHO WANTS CONTROL

"Plans are worthless, but planning is everything."

DWIGHT D. EISENHOWER

*"Setting goals is easy; achieving them is hard. Why?
This question has long stumped humanity."*

ELLIOT T. BERKMAN

The race didn't start until 4 PM, which meant hours of waiting and worrying. I knew I needed to eat, but nothing too heavy. Too much fiber? Bloating. Too much fat? Heavy stomach. Spicy or fried? Risky business. Memories of mid-run vomiting and near bowel catastrophes haunted me.

My mind was running faster than my legs could, calculating blood sugar levels, glycogen stores, and sweat rates. The plan called for a 500-calorie meal before the race. But I wasn't hungry.

Stress had already shut down my digestion. Still, I followed the plan: white rice, chicken, and water—more fuel than food.

As I sat down, I barely noticed the meal. My thoughts were on the course, the heat, and the competition. Bite. Swallow. Repeat. I dumped too much salt on the chicken. Half of it slid into my lap. I brushed it off my legs, unconcerned.

This wasn't eating for survival, pleasure, or socializing. It was eating for performance.

Meet Your Strategic Eater

If you've ever forced a Gatorade down the hatch mid-game or scrutinized nutrition labels in the grocery store aisle, you know this part of yourself. It's the part that meal preps on Sunday nights or calculates whether a late-night snack is "worth it." It's the inner advisor that weighs every food choice against your goals— whether that's losing weight, building muscle, managing choles- terol, or simply feeling more energetic.

This part of you doesn't eat for joy; it eats for results. It analyzes, controls, and optimizes, thinking about food more than experiencing it. In my race-day example above, its mission was crystal clear: Fuel up for thirteen miles of Spartan obstacles without compromising performance. Even though my food was unappetizing and eating was mechanical, I can thank this part for doing its job well. I finished in the top ten in my age bracket, impeccably fueled and hydrated. My success stemmed from a simple yet powerful question: Will eating this help me achieve my goals?

That laser focus is both a gift and a burden of the Strategic Eater. Its logic is clean and measurable, but too much causes rigidity that leaves little room for nuance or intuition. The result, as you're about to discover, is that this member of your eating family can be your greatest ally or your most demanding critic.

Evolutionary Origins:
From Survival to Optimization

Picture your ancestors during a harsh winter. Those who strategically preserved summer's bounty, organized hunting parties, and calculated which plants offered the most nutrition for the least effort had a distinct survival advantage. Strategic eating meant the difference between thriving and starving. As Paul Rozin, the foremost psychologist on food choice, writes: "Securing enough food for survival was a serious challenge ... and given that getting food is a very basic and persistent need, it is not surprising that there has been great evolutionary pressure to develop an efficient foraging system."[1]

That efficient foraging system revolved around thinking about food—where to find it, how to grow it, how to preserve it, and what happened if it ran out. There is even evidence derived from rat studies that mammals have specific neurons which are dedicated to remembering where to find food.[2] Unfortunately, this preoccupation with procuring and storing food can turn into circling the aisles of Costco with a sixty-four pack of muffins you never intended to buy. The challenges of food scarcity that once drove strategic eating have now been replaced by their opposites—the abundance, convenience, and endless choices of a Food 2.0 world.

In response to this new landscape, a new type of Strategic Eater emerged. This one was built on a modern understanding of calories, macronutrients (also known as macros—protein, carbs, fats, and fiber), vitamins, and antioxidants. In the western world, this new way of thinking became enmeshed in nutritionism: the scientific reduction of food to its component parts. Nutritionism transformed food into data to be optimized, rather than sustenance to be enjoyed. Nutritionism ushered in a new era of thinking about food through the lens of achievement, as a means to some other end. Nutrition labels promise us calorie control. Wearable devices offer us precision tracking. Supplements pledge simple solutions to nutrient deficiencies. Metabolic health has become entangled in the complexities of diet culture, biomedical terminology, and modern wellness trends. Contemporary eating has been thoroughly nutrified, quantified, repackaged, and sold alongside a compelling promise: Dial in your macros, find the right supplements, track your metrics, and you'll win the "game" of eating, being rewarded with a fit body and robust health.

We're told the math is foolproof.

Protein = good

Sugar = bad

Calories in < calories out = weight loss

But when you start poking around under the hood, you'll notice nuance and discrepancies that the food, diet, or fitness industry doesn't want you to see. Is more protein universally good? Are all forms of sugar equally bad? Can you perfectly measure and monitor every meal? Is that even desirable?

As we'll find out, there's a lot more uncertainty about how food impacts your mind and body than your Strategic Eater often likes to admit. This doesn't mean we should abandon all hope for metabolically healthy eating, but rather that we need to be judicious about how tightly we hold onto the idea of "quantified health" as the deciding factor in our food choices.

Recognizing the Voice of Your Strategic Eater

Your Strategic Eater typically speaks in the language of goals, data, and meal plans. If your inner dialogue sounds like this, you're probably relying on your Strategic Eater.

- *I need more protein at breakfast to recover from yesterday's workout.*
- *I had a lot of processed carbs for lunch; maybe I should focus on getting more fiber and veggies for dinner.*
- *This restaurant meal looks huge—double what I normally have for lunch—let's save half for later.*
- *Can I make this dish more blood sugar-friendly?*

Or maybe you recognize this part of you in your behaviors when you:

- Check nutrition labels before putting items in your cart.
- Plan tomorrow's meals to balance food groups and nutrients.
- Time your snacks to enhance your workout schedule.
- Feel accomplished for hitting your dietary goals.

For your Strategic Eater, food is a means to achieve something greater. For some, this means training for a marathon. For others, it's simply trying to have more energy for their kids or avoid indigestion that ruins their evening. For others still, it's about aligning their eating habits with personal and planetary well-being. Whether noble or nitpicky, the Strategic Eater's drive is the same: to make every bite serve a larger purpose.

193

The Wisdom of Your Strategic Eater

When it's functioning well, your Strategic Eater provides you with the crisp logic and clear foresight to make informed food choices.

THE GIFT OF INTENTIONALITY IN A FOOD 2.0 WORLD

While your other Inner Eaters tend to live in the moment, your Strategic Eater thinks ahead. It's the part of you that connects today's choices to tomorrow's outcomes.

This long-term perspective is invaluable in a world designed for instant gratification. When every food company is engineering products to trigger immediate pleasure, your Strategic Eater asks the crucial question: *"How will I feel about this choice in an hour? Tomorrow? Next month?"*

This intentionality helps you proactively modify your eating rather than relying on old defaults. Maybe you could eat pizza and beer at midnight in college without consequence, but now, that same meal leaves you bloated, constipated, and sluggish the next day. Perhaps the training diet that fueled your marathon PR doesn't match your current desk job reality. Your Strategic Eater can help you evolve your diet to match who you are now, not who you were a decade ago.

But there's a catch. Your Strategic Eater requires a lot of mental energy to function. When you're stressed, exhausted, or overwhelmed, this goes offline first.[3] That's why building supportive systems matters so much: to give your Strategic Eater the best chance to show up when you need it most.

THE HEALTH STEWARD:
EATING AS MEDICINE AND LONGEVITY

"I need to change my eating, or I'm going to die early," Phil told me after his father passed from heart disease and diabetes complications. Phil's Strategic Eater had awakened with urgent clarity: Every food choice was now a choice about how long he would live.

Sometimes, the doctor delivers the news—type 2 diabetes, cardiovascular disease, IBS, or an autoimmune condition—and suddenly, food takes on new meaning like it did for Phil. What was once just breakfast becomes part of a treatment plan.

In these moments, your Strategic Eater becomes essential. While other parts of you might mourn the loss of favorite foods or worry about social situations where your dietary restrictions cause friction, your Strategic Eater rises to the challenge of using food as medicine. It researches, learns, and adapts to your body's new requirements. In supermarket aisles filled with thousands of engineered food products making exaggerated health claims, your Strategic Eater serves as a translator and watchdog. Whereas your Pleasure Eater reaches for those perfectly moist blueberry muffins, your Strategic Eater quietly asks, *"Should we check what's actually in those muffins?"*

When your Strategic Eater adopts the health steward role, it asks: *"Will this food promote disease?"* It becomes fascinated with:

- **Inflammation and gut health.** *"Are these ingredients irritating my digestion?"*

- **Chemical exposure.** *"What pesticides or additives am I consuming?"*

- **Blood markers.** *"Will this help or hurt my cholesterol, blood pressure, or blood sugar?"*

- **Cellular support.** *"Does this nourish my microbiome or poison it?"*

Your Strategic Eater understands something profound: every bite sends information to trillions of cells in your body. It recognizes that you're nourishing an entire ecosystem of gut bacteria and cellular powerhouses called mitochondria. This awareness transforms eating into an act of biological stewardship, supporting both your microbiome and your cellular energy systems.

For your microbiome, it might urge you to:

- Prioritize a diverse range of plant foods for their varied polyphenols and prebiotics.

- Include fermented foods like yogurt, kimchi, or sauerkraut in your meals.

- Avoid antibiotics, emulsifiers, and artificial additives in ultraprocessed foods.

For your mitochondria, it might suggest:

- Eating with circadian rhythms to optimize your cellular efficiency.

- Consuming vital nutrients like B vitamins, magnesium, and CoQ10.

- Using strategic fasting to trigger cellular renewal.

- Avoiding excess sugar or calorie intake that overwhelms mitochondrial function.

Nourishing these cells is a responsibility that should not be taken lightly. But this approach can go too far. I've seen people create such restrictive "longevity protocols" that food became a source of anxiety for them rather than nourishment. When the pursuit of perfect health becomes an obsession with avoiding death, your Strategic Eater can imprison you in your own good intentions.

The key is how you work with this drive to stay alive and healthy. You can approach any food with fear and rigid restriction, or with curiosity and flexible boundaries. One version of your Strategic Eater is open and accepting of new information; the other is closed off and judgmental. The difference often lies in your conscious leadership. When guided wisely, your Strategic Eater can help you see nutritional realities without becoming neurotic about every unfamiliar ingredient.

THE MEAL PLANNING MAESTRO: CREATING SUSTAINABLE SYSTEMS

If your refrigerator had a project manager, it would be your Strategic Eater. It loves spreadsheets, checklists, and excels at building routines that keep you fed. Every time you've made a grocery list, prepped tomorrow's lunch, or stashed bananas to prevent desperate vending-machine moments, your Strategic Eater was at the helm.

Simplifying dinner decisions, or prepping breakfasts the night before, do more than save time. They preserve your mental energy for what matters most. Your Strategic Eater knows that systems sustain, willpower wanes. Creating supportive routines around grocery shopping and meal planning has upfront costs, but in the long run, they help you conserve energy and avoid impulsive decisions. This is especially powerful for parents who face the additional pressure of feeding themselves and their growing children.

My Strategic Eater shows up every Sunday to map out family dinners for the week ahead. We grocery shop and strategically thaw foods for the meals to come. All of the planning goes onto a

Post-it note stuck to the side of the fridge—Monday: chicken tikka with chickpeas and salad; Tuesday: fish tacos with beans and slaw; Wednesday: DIY (my wife's favorite), and so forth. This way, whenever dinner rolls around, there's no hesitation, confusion, or drama. Consult the Post-it. Dinner is a solved problem.

Planning meals ahead becomes even more powerful when it's paired with observation. Your Strategic Eater can notice patterns of how certain foods affect your energy, mood, digestion, sleep, and overall well-being. For instance, it wants to know the answers to questions like:

- Do you feel more satisfied when you include protein in your breakfast?
- Did those jalapeno-heavy leftovers you ate last night give you heartburn?
- Do you sleep better when you eat dinner earlier?

Insights like these help you fine-tune your meal choices to the evolving needs of your body and life. This is what prevents the preemptive planning from becoming stale. Flexibility is key. What is true today might not be true a month from now. The key is to regularly revisit your meal planning routines to ensure they continue to support you and the needs of your Inner Eaters— Eating 2.0 is not a one-time upgrade!

THE PLANET PROTECTOR: ENVIRONMENTAL AWARENESS

"What's CO_2e?" my wife asked, peering at the lunch menu in the casual Stockholm café. Next to each dish was not a calorie count, as I was used to in some American restaurants, but a climate impact score.

The steak burrito was 3.04 kg CO_2e (high carbon).

The sweet potato burrito was 0.46 kg CO_2e (low carbon)

"We've had carbon labels for about a year," the server explained. "They help people make lower-impact choices."

That moment changed how I thought about my lunch burrito. All of a sudden, my Strategic Eater had an entirely new dimension to consider. It wasn't just concerned with personal health; it was cogitating planetary health.

When your Strategic Eater dons the environmental impact lens, it starts asking new questions, such as:

- *"What chemical fertilizers were used to grow that food?"*
- *"How much fossil fuel was burned to transport these ingredients?"*
- *"Were the farm and factory workers paid a living wage?"*
- *"Is the packaging recyclable or compostable?"*
- *"How much water was wasted or polluted in the process?"*

This perspective recognizes that most of our meals carry invisible costs. A bag of tortilla chips doesn't contain just corn, oil, and salt. It also contains patented monocultures, global transport, unknown labor conditions, and plastic waste.

Our great-grandparents didn't need carbon labels because their food came from *their* land, *their* neighbors, and *their* soil. Today, it comes from everywhere and nowhere, severing the link between eater and eaten—what activist and poet Wendell Berry calls the Industrial Eater: one who does not know that eating is an agricultural act.[4]

This lens may evoke feelings of guilt and moral discomfort. As climate change accelerates and food systems become more fragile, every bite we take is a vote for the world we want to live in. Although you personally had nothing to do with these unsustainable food systems, with this awareness, you are in a position to take action about them.

THE PERFORMANCE OPTIMIZER: FOOD AS PERFORMANCE ENHANCEMENT

Before dawn breaks, Kyle is already up, blending a concoction of kale, blueberries, and protein powder. It's part of his morning routine that is optimized for fuel and nutrients. As a former elite athlete turned high-performing executive, his Strategic Eater treats every meal like part of his performance-enhancing regimen.

Kyle is the poster child for the performance-driven Strategic Eater that turns food into a functional tool for:

- Athletic training and recovery.
- Mental clarity and focus.
- Energy optimization and fatigue prevention.
- Biometric tracking and adjustment.

Tech and science have supercharged this approach. Protein powders, electrolyte blends, and engineered recovery drinks are now standard tools, not just for athletes, but for anyone who aspires to great health and productivity. Continuous glucose monitors, sleep trackers, and genetic food tests give people like Kyle endless data to analyze and optimize their diet.

If you recall the story at the beginning of this chapter, I was leveraging this strength of my Strategic Eater on race day, programming my body with food to win. And for all intents and purposes, it worked. I performed well. No bonk. No vomiting. No regrets.

But here's the catch: When performance becomes everything, the beautiful acts of eating—licking your fingers, dribbling sauce on your chin, scooping an extra-large spoonful because it looks so delicious—become nothing. Food gets reduced to fuel. Input. A checkbox on a productivity spreadsheet. When taken to extremes, this Strategic Eater might prefer engineered nutrition products over shared meals. Huel anyone?

The question becomes: When does the science of high-performance lose the soul of eating? And at what cost?

The Shadow Side of the Strategic Eater: Vulnerabilities and Blind Spots

Your Strategic Eater means well, but like any part of you, it can become hypervigilant, moralistic, and rigid. When it relies too heavily on modern metrics without considering these measures from a holistic point of view, it can lose sight of eating as an embodied experience, casting long shadows of anxiety and fanaticism.

THE OBSESSION TRAP:
WHEN "HEALTHY" EATING TURNS HARMFUL

The most concerning shadow of your Strategic Eater is when the pursuit of perfect eating becomes an obsession. Food stops being nourishment and becomes a source of anxiety. Every meal becomes a test you can pass or fail. Every day is either a tremendous success or a complete failure.

I lived this way for years. I couldn't walk past a bakery without my Strategic Eater launching into lectures about blood sugar and empty calories. I stared at cakes with disbelief that someone would willingly consume so much sugar and fat in one serving. I developed elaborate rules about which foods were "worth it" and which weren't, as if my moral character depended on my relationship

201

with carbohydrates. Once again, these thoughts were remnants of my earlier eating disorder. The line between helpful nutritional discernment and harmful obsession was thin and elusive.

When your Strategic Eater takes over completely, it disconnects from your other Inner Eater's needs. Joy disappears. Intuition vanishes. You become so focused on eating "perfectly" that you lose sight of eating peacefully. You may cling to certain "safe" foods or cut out entire food groups because you think they're unhealthy. This can lead to nutrient deficiencies and other imbalances. Ironically, the very part meant to promote your health can end up harming it—the "cure" worse than the disease.

An extreme fixation with food purity is known as orthorexia nervosa: an unhealthy obsession with "healthy eating." Although orthorexia is not officially recognized as an eating disorder, it captures the anxiety many Americans feel in a food culture where every aisle, influencer, and headline insists on a new "right" way to eat. Modern wellness culture can twist genuine care for the body into a rigid, joyless set of rules that leaves people more stressed than ever. The line between mindful moderation of Food 2.0 and forceful restraint depends on whether your Strategic Eater is a cooperative, balanced part of your Inner Eater family or a rogue despot, demanding compliance. One serves; the other severs.

THE CONTROL TRAP:
WHEN FOOD BECOMES YOUR SAFETY NET

Your Strategic Eater often reaches for control when life feels chaotic—AI threatening to take your job, relationship troubles, natural disasters, economic uncertainty—in these situations, controlling your food can feel like the one thing you can manage. Your Strategic Eater takes advantage of this with a persuasive suggestion: Master food and you master a critical piece of your life.

There is an important truth in that statement. Being extremely disciplined with food can be grounding and empowering. And sometimes, measuring or tracking your food intake genuinely helps you learn about your habits and manage the super-abundance of Food 2.0. Tracking gives clarity on what you've *actually been eating* instead of what you vaguely remember munching on yesterday. For many, this audit is a much-needed reality check.

But when tracking becomes controlling, your Strategic Eater overreaches. It starts promising impossible things like *"If you hit all your protein numbers, you'll lose weight and build muscle"* or *"If you eat completely unprocessed food, you'll never get sick."*

No amount of dietary control can protect you from other people's judgements or life's inherent uncertainty. You can't stop a partner from pulling away emotionally, but your Strategic Eater might double down on counting macros as if precision on a plate could fix what feels uncertain at home. You can't control whether your boss criticizes your presentation, but your Strategic Eater might convince you that skipping dinner will somehow give you back a sense of power.

When your Strategic Eater tries to solve nonfood problems through food control, it creates a fragile system that inevitably breaks down under pressure.

THE ALL-OR-NOTHING TRAP: WHEN NUANCE DISAPPEARS

Your Strategic Eater loves clear categories: good foods versus bad foods, clean eating versus junk food, on-plan versus off-plan. These labels can feel helpful at first—until they become rigid rules that leave no room for imperfection.

Maybe you learned that sugar is "bad," so now you feel guilty about eating fruit. Maybe you read that carbs are "dangerous," so you avoid the pasta at your friend's dinner party. Many of these black-and-white rules stem from insecurities about your body and the food rules in your household. (Return to the chapter on the Social Eater for a deeper dive into generational eating patterns.)

The all-or-nothing trap also arises from sensationalist news and social media posts, where divisive, polarizing, and extreme claims tend to gain the most traction. Perhaps you saw a TikTok that claimed dairy is toxic, so you stopped enjoying the cheese you actually love, even though your body tolerates it just fine. Many questionable food rules get attached to social values about status and worth. The hidden message is that you must not eat "those things" if you want to be healthy.

When you can only see eating in extremes, moderation becomes impossible. Any deviation from the "perfect" plan feels like total failure, often leading to shame and disappointment. Your Strategic Eater's attempt to create safety through rules actually creates more chaos because most eating cannot be easily put into buckets of either "good" or "bad."

THE BODY IMAGE TRAP:
WHEN SELF-WORTH BECOMES SCALE-DEPENDENT

Every year, millions of people attempt to lose weight on a diet. For many, this becomes their default setting. It is so common to diet, in fact, that many people assume that *strategic eating* means cutting calories.

When your Strategic Eater links your body size directly to your worthiness as a person, eating becomes a vehicle for proving you're disciplined, valuable, and lovable, and the scale becomes the judge. The logic goes like this: Control calories in; increase calories out. Become smaller. Become better. *Voilà!* You may now declare yourself "worthy."

This pattern is understandable in a culture that equates body size and shape with everything from virtue to attractiveness to confidence. But it's also a trap with incredibly painful consequences. Your worth isn't determined by what you weigh or whether you are stick-thin or curvy. Regrettably, your Strategic Eater can become obsessed with controlling your body size in order to shape how others see and treat you.

Now, if you've ever lost weight and felt proud of yourself, that's a real accomplishment and worth celebrating. There are definitive social benefits to being in a smaller body: less discrimination, higher salaries, and better medical care, to name a few.[5] Our social systems are biased against big people. It isn't fair, and it isn't right.

The problem isn't that people want to lose weight; it's that research shows that dieting to lose weight often leads to regaining weight (and then some).[6] Weight cycling may promote insulin resistance, dyslipidemia, and even hypertension. More importantly, it perpetuates a system where self-love and self-acceptance depend on external validation. Internal wisdom gets lost when the scale can make or break your day. Even natural weight fluctuations may trigger feelings of failure or inadequacy, prompting your Strategic Eater to take desperate measures to regain control.

Underneath this shadow lie unspoken fears: the fear of getting fat, of being judged, of worsening health. These fears are understandable; however, when your Social Eater turns eating into an anxious transaction of changing body size, rather than an act of caring for the body you currently have, food becomes a battlefield between restriction and rebellion where no one wins.

THE ISOLATION EFFECT:
WHEN FOOD RULES DAMAGE RELATIONSHIPS

An overactive Strategic Eater can slowly separate you from the people and experiences you value. Eating out with friends? Too many calories. Family holiday traditions? Too many unhealthy dishes. Restaurant dates? No control over ingredients.

At first, these choices might feel empowering—you're prioritizing your health goals. If you typically overeat or never set appropriate boundaries at social meals, this represents a shift toward conscious consumption and greater self-determination. However, what starts as a quest for health can slowly morph into loneliness. This is an issue of integration, finding the sweet spot between your Strategic Eater's goals and your Social Eater's needs for human connection.

THE BIGGER PICTURE YOUR STRATEGIC EATER MISSES

Your Strategic Eater's limitations are a natural consequence of having a mind-over-matter perspective. This aspect of you excels at *thinking about food*, but underperforms in the realm of embodied awareness or sensory appreciation. As a result, cognitive biases and distortions silently shape your food decisions.

Your Strategic Eater can draft the perfect eating plan, but it struggles with:

- **All-or-nothing thinking.** *I had a cookie, so I blew it—may as well order pizza.*

- **Confirmation bias.** Selectively noticing articles, posts, or anecdotes that support your chosen eating plan (*See, another study proves seed oils are evil!*) while ignoring evidence or personal experiences that contradict it.

- **Metric fixation.** For example, pursuing an objective like restricting yourself to 1,800 calories or consuming 150 grams of protein daily while overlooking qualitative factors such as stress, taste, and fullness.

- **Moral licensing.** *I worked out and ate a salad, so I earned this milkshake.*

- **Authority bias.** Overvaluing the opinions of a particular "guru" or influencer because of credentials/charisma rather than how their advice fits with your body and lifestyle.

When you zoom out and look at the broader Food 2.0 landscape, it demands the discernment of your Strategic Eater. However, peaceful and purposeful eating requires more than strategy alone. It requires integration of all your needs, many of which can't be quantified or captured by data or logic alone. This is the lesson your Strategic Eater has yet to learn: No system map, no diet plan, and no amount of tracking can fully account for the complex emotional undercurrents of eating in a Food 2.0 world. Only the conscious leader within you can hold the full complexity of your eating without getting lost in egotistical illusions.

Your Strategic Eater's Personal History

Sometimes your Strategic Eater springs to life from a health scare that makes avoiding certain foods medically necessary. Other times, it emerges from cultural messages about productivity, worth, or perfection. However it formed, your Strategic Eater has an origin story. And when you understand that story, you gain the power to work with it more skillfully, rather than letting it run the show in the background.

It's possible your Strategic Eater emerged from positive influences: parents who meal-planned thoughtfully, involvement in sports that sparked curiosity about nutrition, or health classes that taught you about food systems and human metabolism. These experiences can create a Strategic Eater that serves you well—a way of thinking about food that's organized, informed, and balanced.

Conversely, your Strategic Eater may have developed from more complicated experiences, such as living in a household obsessed with dieting, or being surrounded by family members constantly commenting on "good" foods and "bad" bodies. You may have been bombarded by weight loss messaging and fatphobic ideas that made your body never seem good enough. This can create a Strategic Eater that's hypervigilant and anxious, always calculating or restricting.

But here's a little catch: not everyone develops a strong Strategic Eater. Maybe no one in your family cared about nutrition, or you never received much education about how food affects your body. Perhaps food decisions were always based on convenience, tradition, or what was available. If you grew up outside the United States, you may not have been exposed to a scientific reductionist approach to food or wellness influencer culture. If you're young and healthy, you may never have to think strategically about the quality or quantity of food you eat.

Developing a strong Strategic Eater requires certain privileges: stable food environments, education, time to plan and shop thoughtfully, and access to diverse food options—forms of privilege that not everyone has access to. Eating "strategically" changes meaning entirely if you're living in a food desert or stretching a tight budget. The goal shifts from optimization to survival and sufficiency. The Strategic Eater of a single parent working multiple jobs may be very blended with their Social or

Survival Eater: thinking about what's cheap and convenient for the whole family, not what this meal can do to further personal or planetary health.

MY STRATEGIC EATER'S DANGEROUS BEGINNING

My own Strategic Eater emerged during the chaos of my teenage years: a changing body, a new high school, rising self-consciousness, and a desperate need to feel in control of something. The more confused I became about who I was—and who I thought I should be—the more fraught my relationship with food became.

What started as curiosity about nutrition quickly became an obsession. I memorized nutrition labels, devoured fitness magazines, and could calculate the macros of any packaged food in seconds. Friends turned it into a party game, showing me a brand and asking me to guess their nutritional stats. I could break down its calories like a contestant on Jeopardy.

My Strategic Eater became powerful—in many ways, too powerful. I could restrict calories with clinical precision, tracking every bite while my body slowly broke down. What felt like expertise became self-destruction in disguise.

That period of my life nearly destroyed me. But I eventually learned to balance my Strategic Eater with the wisdom of my other Inner Eaters, integrating it as a source of strength rather than of suffering.

Your Strategic Eater's story might be completely different from mine. (In many ways, I hope it is.) Maybe this part never got hung up on counting, scrutinizing, and double-checking food. Maybe it's absent, but you're working to strengthen it. Maybe it's overactive and needs to learn to step back. Whatever the case may be, the next section will help you better consciously lead your Strategic Eater so you can navigate the world of Food 2.0 with resilience, not rigidity.

Leading Your Strategic Eater Wisely

What counts as strategic isn't the same for everyone—and it won't stay the same across your lifespan. In different seasons, your Strategic Eater will highlight different priorities, sometimes subtly, sometimes dramatically. A middle-aged parent might prioritize weight loss. Someone managing diabetes might focus on eating for longevity. An athlete will likely emphasize performance and recovery. An avid gardener may center their choices on plant-based foods grown close to home.

The goal isn't to pick the "right" version of strategy. The goal is awareness of which lens your Strategic Eater is currently using, and then relating to this part with CARE instead of letting it operate unconsciously in the background.

CURIOSITY:
UNDERSTANDING YOUR STRATEGIC EATER'S PATTERNS

Start by getting curious about how your Strategic Eater shows up in your life: Is it overdeveloped—rigid, anxious, obsessed with goals? Is it underdeveloped—absent, vague, uninterested in planning? Both extremes deserve your attention.

If your Strategic Eater runs the show. Maybe every bite feels calculated and every meal becomes overanalyzed. You might recognize thoughts like *I must track everything perfectly* or *I ate too much fat earlier. I'll eat nonfat the rest of the day.* Without reflection, it's hard to know if this is coming from a place of wisdom or shadow. You need to ask yourself: *Is this serving me as a conscious leader or feeding the anxiety of an overactive Strategic Eater?*

If it is coming from a fearful place inside, consider what this part is trying to protect you from. Fear of losing control? Worry about health? A need to feel safe in an uncertain world?

Take out a piece of paper and a pen and write down what comes up. Don't try to fix it, just notice it.

If Your Strategic Eater has gone silent. Sometimes this voice disappears entirely, and you don't even realize it until it comes time to dine and intention is nowhere to be found. Planning meals may feel overwhelming or irrelevant. Mindless eating or drinking may be too easy and too ingrained. Perhaps you don't even know where to begin thinking more critically about food.

Instead of feeling embarrassed, get curious. Ask yourself:

- *If my Strategic Eater focused on "good enough for now," what choice would it make?*

- *What's the cost of not thinking ahead about my meals?*

- *If my Strategic Eater is totally silent, who is making my food choices?*

Curiosity isn't about forcing yourself to become a meal planner; it's about understanding what gets in the way of a more proactive approach to eating.

APPRECIATION:
HONORING THIS VOICE'S CONTRIBUTIONS

Your Strategic Eater has likely done more for you than you give it credit for, quietly steering you toward healthier options, supporting your efforts to build strength, and reminding you to eat in ways that sustain your energy over the long haul. Take a moment to acknowledge this. Say: *I appreciate how you keep me on track. I see the work you do to help me think ahead and make intentional choices.*

When you acknowledge your Strategic Eater's positive intentions, you reduce its need to fight for control. Gratefulness helps it relax, releasing its need to be the sole guardian of your well-being.

RESPONSIBILITY: TAKE OWNERSHIP OF YOUR CHOICES

Once your Strategic Eater feels seen and valued, you can invite it to take its rightful place as one helpful voice among many, instead of the only one calling the shots. You get to decide when to follow its guidance and when to push back.

The next time you catch yourself in automatic rule-following or deferring to external authority, pause and reframe whatever you're thinking to make it a personal choice. For example, instead of skipping an espresso martini after dinner because you've been told there's too many calories or too much caffeine, try replacing "I should" with "I choose to." For instance, *I choose to skip drinking tonight because I am the type of person who cares about my health.* Or, *I choose to have the birthday cake because connection with my friends matters more than perfect nutrition right now.*

This approach:

- Maintains your agency rather than solely relying on external expectations.

- Honors your Strategic Eater's concerns without being controlled by them.

- Acknowledges every choice has tradeoffs—the key is making them consciously.

- Prevents resentment by owning your choices fully.

EXPLORATION:
EXPANDING BEYOND RIGID PATTERNS

Your Strategic Eater loves control, but growth often requires leaning into uncertainty. One way to practice is through small experiments, intentionally stepping outside your usual habits, then observing what actually happens. By testing instead of assuming, you help your Strategic Eater discover that uncertainty is a chance to learn.

For example, if you:

- Always track calories, then try eating one meal based purely on intuition and satisfaction.

- Never plan meals, then experiment with preparing tomorrow's lunch the night before.

- Avoid certain foods altogether, then try them in a small amount and notice what actually happens in your mouth and body.

- Eat the same breakfast every day, then try something different and observe how you feel afterward.

Frame these as time-bound experiments rather than permanent changes. It's not, "We are going to eat this way forever." It's, "Let's try this for a few days and see what happens." Your Strategic Eater can get on board with gathering data and testing assumptions if it knows there's a definitive endpoint. Committing to a specific number of meals or days also makes it easier to commit and stay accountable for following through.

The beauty of loosening your rules, even slightly, is that you may uncover assumptions that were never true. Just beyond your Strategic Eater's comfort zone often lies more satisfying and sustainable eating than you imagined. The question is whether you're willing to let go of control to regain choice.

Looking Ahead:
From Control to Collaboration

Your Strategic Eater is essential for navigating Food 2.0's misleading marketing and irresistible treats, but we must not forget Eisenhower's wisdom that opens the chapter: "Plans are worthless, but planning is everything." Your Strategic Eater's real gift is the process of thoughtful consideration itself—the planning, the reflecting, the intentional thinking about how food serves your life. This matters far more than rigid adherence to any specific set of rules.

When you lead your Strategic Eater wisely, it provides clarity and structure without becoming controlling. It thinks ahead and then eases up so you don't lose touch with what's happening right now. This is where your Strategic Eater's planning works best, when it's informed by your Pleasure Eater's enjoyment, your Social Eater's need for connection, and your Survival Eater's guardianship of your body.

Now that you're familiar with the four major parts of your eating family, the journey of eating evolves from trying to manage each inner part separately to learning how to lead them all together. This is what we'll tackle in Part Three. You'll learn how to consistently step into the role of the conscious leader—the part that can wisely hold space for all your different Inner Eaters—and navigate Food 2.0 challenges in real-world eating scenarios.

PART III
THE EATING 2.0 UPGRADE

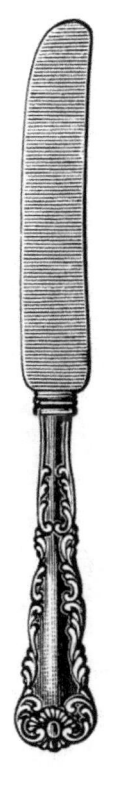

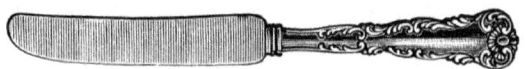

NINE

INNER LEADERSHIP

TAKING THE SEAT AT THE HEAD OF YOUR OWN TABLE

"All leaders must have two things: They must have a vision of the world that does not exist and they must have the ability to communicate it."

SIMON SINEK

The sun rose at 6:37 AM, and by 6:52, James was already behind schedule. A senior product manager at a major software company, James lived with his wife, Melissa, a freelance graphic designer, and their three-year-old daughter in a townhouse outside Seattle. Like many dual-career couples with a young child, their days were packed. Between early meetings, daycare drop-off, and the constant juggling act of modern parenting, food often became an afterthought.

Standing in his kitchen, James grabbed supplies while mentally rehearsing his day. Two yogurts sat in the fridge: one loaded with caramel and fruit, the other plain. His Strategic Eater flickered to life— *"This one's probably has less sugar"* —as he reached for the plain version. He ate it standing up while checking emails, yogurt dribbling down his chin as his mind raced ahead to work deadlines.

The reality was James hadn't enjoyed a meal in months, not truly. Every bite came at a breakneck speed while he was doing something else. He'd gained fifteen pounds since becoming a dad, in part because he never really paid attention to how much he was eating. Meals became makeshift moments, cobbling together whatever seemed the most tasty or easiest. Sometimes, that meant his dinner and eating the leftovers on his daughter's plate as well. Despite having more than enough food, he was constantly hungry, or at least felt like he could always eat—the cruel irony of Food 2.0 overstimulating our appetites.

On the short drive to his office, James passed Starbucks, already buzzing with the morning crowd. He saw people walking out of the store clutching large coffee drinks and paper-wrapped breakfast sandwiches. James's Pleasure Eater stirred for just a moment— *"Maybe I should stop for one of those delicious breakfast sandwiches too"* —but his Strategic Eater quickly shut it down: *"Just keep driving, you already ate."* So, he did, though the craving lingered, unresolved.

By noon, stress and boredom had taken over. James found himself at the office fridge, staring at leftover pizza beside a neglected bed of lettuce that once resembled a salad. He peeked at the pizza. Sausage and onion, his favorite. His Pleasure Eater urged him to heat it up, but he scarfed it down cold, straight from the box.

That evening, James and Melissa had planned to cook salmon together—a moment of connection they'd both been looking forward to. But after a long day and their daughter's meltdown, James stared at the fresh ingredients and felt overwhelmed. "Not tonight," he informed his wife, "I don't have it in me." Instead, they ate separately. For his meal, he reheated leftover Thai food, eating at the counter while dipping fresh spring rolls in sauce and scrolling through his phone. He probably would have eaten the entire container, but his Social Eater looked up from his phone and thought for a moment to save some for Melissa.

Later, eyeing his daughter's leftover brownie, James felt caught between conflicting drives: *I want that* versus *It's not a good idea.* After what had already been a long day, James was now stuck in this internal tug-of-war, feeling full yet unsatisfied. Clearly, something was "off," but he couldn't quite name it.

What Happens Without a Conscious Leader

James hadn't eaten poorly, exactly. But he hadn't eaten in a way that felt aligned with the man he wanted to be. What was missing wasn't willpower or nutrition knowledge—it was leadership. Without conscious leadership, James's day became a series of handoffs between his different Inner Eaters, each reacting to immediate pressures without considering the bigger picture.

If we analyze Jame's day, the stages were as follows.

Morning rush. His Survival Eater grabbed the easiest option— yogurt—with a cameo from his Strategic Eater: *"Choose the one without caramel sauce. It's probably healthier."*

Drive to work. His Strategic Eater overruled his Pleasure Eater's Starbucks desire. *"Just keep driving."*

Lunch break. His Pleasure Eater got the salty, savory pizza it was craving, but not exactly the way it wanted—he ate it cold, straight out of the box.

Dinner time. His Survival Eater chose convenience over his Social Eater's plan to cook and connect with his wife.

219

Evening. All his parts started arguing over the brownie, leaving him dissatisfied and internally torn up.

This result is what you might expect from leaving unsupervised children in charge of a kitchen. Each Inner Eater has valid needs, but without coordination from a leader, you get chaos: cold pizza, abandoned plans, and lots of frustration.

The consequences of this leaderless eating extend far beyond individual meals. When your Inner Eaters constantly fight for control, it creates:

- **Physical stress.** Irregular eating patterns, mindless consumption, and poor food choices that may compound into fatigue, digestive issues, or inflammation.

- **Mental exhaustion.** The constant internal negotiation drains energy that could be used for other important parts of your life.

- **Emotional frustration.** Repeatedly falling short of your own intentions creates a cycle of disappointment and self-criticism.

Our Food 2.0 environment makes conscious leadership genuinely difficult. It's hard to choose well when you are stressed out, riled up, and overactivated—chasing a sugar high, literally and metaphorically.

But here's what's important: You have more power than you realize. While you can't get rid of the challenges of living in a Food 2.0 world, you can learn to lead your Inner Eaters more skillfully.

What Inner Leadership Actually Looks Like

Most of us try to manage our eating like bad bosses manage people—through control, rigid rules, and forced compliance. But there's a profound difference between being a boss and being a conscious leader.

Bosses ask: "Are we following the rules?"
Leaders ask: "What do we actually need right now?"

Bosses impose control.
Leaders provide direction.

Bosses react to problems.
Leaders create possibilities.

With your Inner Eaters, the boss approach looks a lot like an overactive Strategic Eater imposing strict food rules and trying to force compliance with through harsh criticism.

Conscious leadership looks different: It involves setting a clear vision, building trust between your Inner Eaters, and creating conditions where each one can contribute its strengths while compensating for its limitations.

True leadership, as my colleague at the Harvard Graduate School of Education, Able Cano, puts it, is "enabling others to achieve a shared purpose in the face of uncertainty."[1]

Conscious Leadership in Action: James's Day Reimagined

Let's rewind James's morning and see what conscious leadership could have looked like. Instead of rushing through his routine in a mindless fog, imagine James pausing for just a moment to ask himself: *Who's hungry right now? What kind of day do "we" want to create together?*

This simple question shifts everything. Instead of letting the loudest Inner Eater take control, James could have taken the seat at the head of his inner table. What would the same decision points have looked like had he led his Inner Eaters?

Morning leadership. Standing in the kitchen with two yogurts, James could have listened to both his Strategic Eater (*"Choose the plain one for better nutrition"*) and his Survival Eater (*"We need fuel fast"*). He could have acknowledged his Survival Eater's urgency: *"I know you feel hurried, but we're not actually in a big rush."* Instead of eating while juggling his daughter's backpack, he might have said to himself: *Okay, let's take sixty seconds to actually pay attention while eating. Maybe I can add some berries we have in the fridge for my Strategic Eater's peace of mind.*

These small adjustments—sitting down, adding fruit, being present for a minute—represent a shift from unconscious reaction to conscious choice.

The coffee shop moment. Driving past Starbucks, instead of just pushing down his Pleasure Eater's craving, James could have gotten curious. *What's really happening here? What am I actually hungry for?*

Did part of him just want to delay arriving in the office? Maybe. Perhaps the thought was less about the bacon and eggs and more about his Pleasure Eater craving novelty. Yogurt from the fridge, boring. A dozen types of breakfast sandwiches, delightful. It's also possible his Social Eater was longing to partake in the coffee shop ritual he saw by joining the morning crowd.

By acknowledging these desires without immediately reacting to them, James could have brought awareness to his previously unconscious parts, preventing them from erupting later in the day as rebellion.

Lunch leadership. At the office fridge, instead of mindlessly grabbing cold pizza, as a leader, he could have paused to reflect,

I'm hungry and bored, but what does my body need here? Energy? Water? A real break from work?

From a place of awareness, James would've had choices he didn't have before. For example, he could have:

- Made a proper plate with pizza and some salad.

- Asked a colleague to sit outside with him for a few minutes of human connection while he ate.

- Taken a small bite to ease his hunger, then made a clearer decision about what would come next.

There's endless adjacent possibilities that integrate his Inner Eaters and help move them towards a shared purpose. Exploring any one of them would have been a move toward lunch leadership.

Dinner decisions. When the evening plans fell apart and exhaustion set in, leadership might have meant asking, *How can I give all my Inner Eaters something they need right now?*

He could have simplified the meal, throwing the salmon in the oven with minimal prep. He could have eaten the Thai leftovers but plated them more thoughtfully and eaten them with his wife instead of standing alone at the counter, scrolling through his phone.

The brownie moment. That final encounter with his daughter's leftover brownie wasn't really about the brownie; it was about a pattern of ending his night with eating more than he wanted. This small but repeated act became a nightly ritual that undermined James's larger intentions. Instead of closing the day with a sense of agency, alignment, and pride, he reinforced the very identity he wanted to move beyond. James, in a leadership role, could have listened to what each voice inside him was saying.

- **Survival Eater:** *"I'm worn out and eating will help me relax."*

- **Pleasure Eater:** *"I want that rich, chocolatey, gooey taste in my mouth."*

223

- **Social Eater:** *"This is something my daughter made. Eating it will be a sign that I appreciate her. Or maybe I should wait and share it with the family."*

- **Strategic Eater:** *"That much fat and sugar before bed is going to sit like a rock in my stomach and mess with my sleep."*

If James had stepped into conscious leadership, he wouldn't have been ruled by any single Inner Eater. Instead, he would have taken responsibility for how to respond to each one. By paying attention to the deeper messages behind their urges, he might have recognized that he really was craving relief from a long day, a sense of connection, and experiencing the pull of hyperpalatable food manipulating his appetite.

The Art of Conscious Tradeoffs

Here's what's crucial to understand: Leadership of your Inner Eaters isn't about making "perfect" food choices—no such thing exists. It's about staying alert to subtle signals, adjusting in real time, and making conscious tradeoffs so that your food choices align with your values and circumstances.

Sometimes, you may prioritize pleasure over strategy, connection over ideal nutrition, or survival over any other consideration. Your needs shift daily, and so should your food choices. When these choices reflect your values and shared purpose rather than your autopilot, you're steering the ship. This is the difference between leading with chosen priorities and following reactive defaults.

As a conscious leader, what might James have done with that brownie he wanted to eat?

- Maybe he would've taken a few thoughtful bites and decided that was enough—no guilt, no regret.

- Maybe he'd have said, "No thanks," and walked away, knowing he could always have it later if he wanted.

- Maybe he'd have waited for his wife and asked if she wanted to share it, turning a solitary moment into an opportunity for connection.

- Maybe he would've eaten the whole thing consciously, taking full responsibility for how it would affect his sleep and energy, without justification or self-criticism.

Any of these choices could have represented conscious leadership, depending on what James and his Inner Eaters needed in that moment. The important part is choosing from a place of clarity and care.

Deepening CARE:
The Four "Muscles" of Conscious Leadership

You've already learned the principles of CARE: using curiosity, appreciation, responsibility, and exploration as the foundation for leading your Inner Eaters. But when you're exhausted, stressed, or overwhelmed, your nervous system could be too activated to access the pillars of CARE.

That's where these four leadership "muscles" come in. Think of them as the internal strengths that make CARE possible, even when life gets chaotic and your wise leadership seems distant. These muscles don't replace CARE; they give you the capacity to put CARE in action.

MUSCLE 1. STORYTELLER VISION:
THE FOUNDATION FOR CURIOSITY

When one Inner Eater takes over, your awareness narrows around a single need—control, relief, pleasure, approval, whatever it may be. In that moment, you become the part, losing sight of the bigger picture.

Storyteller Vision is the ability to zoom out and see the whole system: all your Inner Eaters, your future self, and your deeper values. It's the shift from living inside one story to becoming the storyteller who decides which story gets airtime.

But here's the catch: you can't access Storyteller Vision when your nervous system is stuck in a stress response. Before you can sit in the storyteller's seat at the head of the table, you need a reset.

KEY PRACTICE:
THE THREE-BREATH RESET

Take three conscious breaths, feeling your belly expand in all directions. Make each exhale slower than your inhale. Let your spine lengthen, shoulders release, and feet anchor firmly on the ground.

Say silently: *I am not just one part. I am the one who sees all parts. I am not the story. I am the storyteller.*

After three conscious breaths, ask: *Am I calm and clear enough to lead wisely right now?*

If the answer is no, try one of these physical resets.

- Continue the three-breath reset as long as needed to regain composure.

- Drink a glass of water and rub your hands together until you feel some warmth.
- Step outside. Look up at the sky, trees, and clouds. Feel the fresh air on your face. Remember you are a part of a much bigger world.
- Shake it out, stretch your body or change positions. For instance, if sitting, stand. If standing, lay down.

From James's day: When James drove past the coffee shop, he might have paused at the red light. Taken three breaths. Then inquired, *Whose story am I living right now?*

He might have noticed his Pleasure Eater wanting something delightful, his Social Eater drawn to the ritual of morning coffee shop culture, his Strategic Eater evaluating nutrition, and his Survival Eater feeling the tug of growing hunger.

MUSCLE 2. RADICAL ACCEPTANCE: THE GATEWAY TO APPRECIATION

We are wired to resist what we don't like—to fight it, deny it, or judge it. But genuine appreciation requires acceptance first.

Acceptance doesn't mean liking everything you notice. It means you stop fighting with reality long enough to understand what's truly going on. When you label your cravings as frustrations or make hunger "wrong," you lose the ability to work with them skillfully.

As meditation teacher Tara Brach says in her book *Radical Acceptance,* "The boundary to what we can accept is the boundary to our freedom."[2]

KEY PRACTICE: "THIS IS TRUE RIGHT NOW"

Place a hand on your heart. Feel your chest rise as you breathe, and your heart beating.

Say: "This is true right now. It may feel uncomfortable, but it will change."

Then ask: "Can I allow this to be what it is, even if it's uncomfortable, confusing, or messy?"

From James's day: Standing before his daughter's brownie after a long, tiring day. James might have placed a hand on his heart and acknowledged, *This is true right now: I both want this brownie and I'm concerned about eating it. Both feelings can exist at the same time.*

James first needs to accept that he's torn before he can appreciate his Strategic Eater's concern for his well-being.

MUSCLE 3. DROPPING DEFENSIVENESS: THE PATH TO RESPONSIBILITY

Conscious leadership requires humility. When we're busy defending, justifying, or making excuses, we forfeit our ability to truly listen. First we need to stop talking. Then we need to own our role in creating the situation we're in, even if it's painful to acknowledge.

This isn't easy. In fact, it may be a lesson of many lifetimes. When you can own your part without defending it, you gain the power to change it.

KEY PRACTICE:
THE ACCOUNTABILITY QUESTION

When you notice defensiveness rising in you, ask yourself: *What part of this situation am I responsible for? How can I own the impact of my words or actions without arguing my point?*

Answer honestly, without adding qualifiers or "but" statements.

Say: *When I did ___, I can imagine the impact would have been . . .*

If needed, add, *Although that wasn't my best move, I can learn from it.*

Complete the sentence: "Next time, I will . . . [fill in the blank]."

From James's day: After scarfing down cold pizza while standing at the office fridge, James might have thought, *I had no choice. I was between meetings and "starving."* Instead, with this practice, he could have asked: *What part of this situation am I responsible for?*

His honest answer would have been, *I'm responsible for not protecting my schedule to make time for lunch, for not paying attention to the food as I was eating, and for not checking in with what I actually wanted.*

Dropping defensiveness clears the way for responsibility. *Next time, I will take at least five minutes to clear my head and determine what my Inner Eaters need before I grab something to eat.* No shame, just well-defined responsibility and a path forward.

MUSCLE 4. EMBRACING UNCERTAINTY: THE SPACE FOR EXPLORATION

Traditional meal planning is built on the illusion that you can know exactly what you'll want, need, or be able to do on Thursday night. It aims to eliminate uncertainty, reduce risk, and minimize the likelihood of being unprepared, all of which are valid and important benefits, for sure. But what do you do when your hunger surprises you, your schedule shifts, or your cravings change? Can you adapt without panic?

The more you embrace uncertainty, the more you can experiment with new ways of relating to your Inner Eaters. Steady routines and predictable meal structures are like steady anchors— use them when you can. But real breakthroughs in eating well often come from disruptions that push you outside your comfort zone and force you to see success differently. You can't discover new ways of eating if you demand certainty about the outcomes. Clarity often comes after an unexpected scramble to get fed. The lesson is to make a plan, but don't cling to it so tightly that you lose the ability to listen and respond to the moment.

KEY PRACTICE: THE PIVOT PLAN

When plans start to unravel, situations shift, and your hunger isn't as predictable as you thought, ask: *Can I be okay with my needs changing?*

Try saying: *This moment is unique. Let's see what works best right now.* This is your chance to take conscious leadership and embrace uncertainty. Even if you can't know exactly what you'll need later, you can stay present enough to meet your Inner Eaters wisely. Anchor in your bigger purpose (recall your values from Chapter 4) and pick the next workable step that balances your needs as best as you can.

From James's day: When James and Melissa's salmon dinner got derailed due to exhaustion and their daughter's meltdown, James saw only two options: Either cook the elaborate meal or abandon it entirely. With Embracing Uncertainty, he might have paused, regulated, and been better able to adjust on the fly. Instead of seeing it in all-or-nothing terms, he could've seen it as feedback or a chance to get creative—simplifying the recipe, pulling together a quick snack plate, or even turning dinner into a family picnic night on the living room floor. By shifting out of panic and into leadership, James could ask not only *What can I learn for next time?* but also *How can I meet my family's needs here and now?*

HOW THESE FOUR MUSCLES WORK TOGETHER

The beauty of these four capacities lies in how they support one another. Storytelling Vision helps you self-regulate so you can see the bigger picture. Radical Acceptance lets you work with reality as it is, not as you wish it to be. Dropping Defensiveness enables you to own every choice, even if it's a hard one. Embracing Uncertainty keeps you flexible enough to improv, adapt, and discover what will work best right now.

Don't worry about building all four capacities at once. Start where you are and strengthen one or two leadership muscles at a time. In a stressful, reactive day, practicing a few conscious breaths to support your Storyteller Vision is progress. A single instance of Dropping Defensiveness, rather than reacting with justification, is growth. All these little moments add up, helping you eat with intention, not by default.

THE FOUR CONSCIOUS LEADERSHIP "MUSCLES"		
Leadership Muscle	CARE Quality	Key Practice
Storyteller Vision	Curiosity	Three-Breath Reset
Radical Acceptance	Appreciation	"This is true right now."
Drop Defensiveness	Responsibility	Accountability Question
Embrace Uncertainty	Exploration	The Pivot Plan

Looking Ahead:
From Inner Leadership to Outer Mastery

Mastering these four muscles of conscious leadership doesn't automatically change your eating habits, but it does enable you to lead, grow, and relate to yourself in wiser and wiser ways. The more you strengthen these capacities, the easier it is to CARE for your Inner Eaters, and the more you can trust yourself to show up in any unexpected situation and make smart, sensible food choices.

As powerful as this inner work is, it doesn't happen in a vacuum. Your ability to lead your Inner Eaters will always be shaped by the environment around you. And today, that environment is not neutral. That's why strong inner leadership must be paired with outer mastery.

In the next chapter, we'll focus on the outer structures, daily habits, and practical systems that either support your Inner Eaters or sabotage them. We'll explore how to design an environment where your conscious leadership can flourish and why Food 2.0 requires new rules of engagement.

TEN

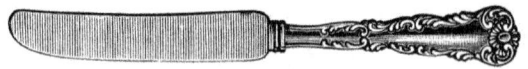

OUTER MASTERY

THE FIVE POWER MOVES FOR EATING 2.0

"1. Research your own experience.
2. Absorb what is useful.
3. Reject what is useless.
4. Add what is specifically your own."

BRUCE LEE, PARAPHRASED BY JOHN LITTLE

You don't get to choose how or when your Inner Eaters show up. They arrive unannounced, sometimes at the worst times, sometimes all at once. That's why the inner work of Eating 2.0 matters so much: It teaches you how to respond to your natural impulses with intense curiosity and strong leadership rather than control or collapse.

But here's the reality: When you're hungry, exhausted, and surrounded by Food 2.0 engineered to hijack your instincts, you won't always rise to your highest leadership potential. In those moments, you'll fall to the level of your systems. This is why it is so important to structure your world to invite your Inner Eater's gifts forward and make reactive choices less likely.

Morning Leadership: Setting the Stage

Let's return to James from the previous chapter, now practicing conscious leadership. He wakes up and asks his familiar question: *What kind of day do we want to create together?* But today he adds: *How can I set up my food environment to support all my Inner Eaters?*

Standing at the open fridge with two yogurts, that's when it hits him—his wife went grocery shopping with their daughter, and of course, they bought the yogurts they enjoy. His own nutritional needs never made it onto the list. In that moment, James sees the larger pattern: without his involvement, his food environment will always be shaped by other people's preferences or by Food 2.0 marketing. Outer mastery means stepping up and taking responsibility for what enters the house in the first place. If he wants his Strategic Eater supported, he needs to join the grocery trips or at least create a list that reflects his needs and goals.

Recognizing that it's his job to curate a space that supports his Inner Eaters, he moves some apples from the crisper drawer to the counter. He also tucks a bag of goldfish crackers deeper into the pantry. Nothing is forbidden, but if his Survival Eater takes over later in the day, he's designed his default to support his larger vision and shared purpose.

System Failures—and Fixes—at Lunch

At noon, when James finds himself in the office kitchen, eyeing leftover sausage pizza, he realizes he didn't pack lunch again. However, this isn't about personal blame; the office kitchen is part of the Food 2.0 environment, full of defaults that push him toward convenience and away from his values.

This is where the outer game matters most. If James had prepared even a simple backup—some leftover dinner, a quick grain bowl, or an easy wrap—he'd have more choices now. He could still eat the pizza if he wanted, but it wouldn't be his only option.

This decision isn't about restriction vs. freedom; it's about preparation. While looking at the pizza, James realizes he needs systems to make conscious leadership easier, so he plans in the future to:

- Pack leftovers the night before.

- Prep a few grab-and-go foods on Sunday.

- Stock the office kitchen with backup options, such as hard-boiled eggs, canned salmon, and premade salad kits.

These become small moves that make his lunches less vulnerable to eating someone else's leftovers or relying on Food 2.0 defaults. They tilt the environment back in his favor, giving him more choices that align with his intentions when hunger strikes.

Dinner:
When Good Intentions Meet Reality

It is now evening, and the ingredients for James's planned teriyaki salmon dinner sit untouched—raw fish, whole vegetables, and uncooked grains. This isn't the first time fresh ingredients have gone unused. Modern life rarely gives him the time and bandwidth to cook from scratch on a weeknight. This is part of Food 2.0's sleight of hand, pushing people towards ultraprocessed foods that make scratch cooking seem too labor intensive.

But here's a pivot he can make in the future: Instead of abandoning home-cooked meals entirely, James could reshape his environment by choosing "strategic convenience" —pre-marinated proteins, bagged salad mixes, precut vegetables, or even a meal kit service with prepped components. Perhaps he could leverage a "halfway homemade" approach by purchasing sides from the market on his way home and cooking a dish at home. All of these would be intentional upgrades, using modern convenience to serve a larger goal: making family dinners possible again.

The Brownie Decision:
Inner Leadership Meets Outer Design

When a brownie appears at day's end, instead of asking *Should I eat this?* Eating 2.0 invites a deeper question: *What kind of eater am I becoming?*

This reframes the moment as part of James's ongoing relationship with food rather than a single "good" or "bad" choice. He applies his Food 2.0 filter: *Is this engineered to be irresistible, effortless, and endless? If so, what pitfalls might arise?*

- **Irresistible**: Yup, the brownie is rich, sweet, and nostalgic.

- **Effortless**: Yup, it's ready to melt in his mouth.

- **Endless**: Nope, this is the last piece.

James recognizes how these three qualities can hijack his Inner Eaters, leading to mindless overconsumption. But outer leadership doesn't mean throwing the brownie away or eating the whole thing. It means putting systems in place so that choices feel more conscious in the moment.

Jame decided to place a small sticky note on the fridge that read: *Irresistible. Effortless. Endless. Lead consciously.* When he saw the note before reaching for the brownie, it reminded him to slow down and decide with intention. Sometimes that pause leads to savoring the brownie fully; other times it leads to skipping it. Either way, he's practicing leadership, not reacting on autopilot.

The Five Power Moves for Eating 2.0: Building the New Default

If you want to help your Inner Eaters thrive, you need to intentionally restore what Food 2.0 systematically removes.

What Food 2.0 removes or minimizes:

- **Fiber.** The natural bulk that feeds your microbiome and signals *"You've had enough."*

- **Micronutrients and phytochemicals.** Critical compounds your body uses to fight inflammation, detoxify, and maintain cellular health.

- **Chewing.** The pause and effort that slow you down and naturally create a sense of satisfaction.

- **Presence.** The fragmented busyness of modern life pulls your attention away from your food and your body.

What Food 2.0 adds:

- **Sugar, salt, and refined fats.** Engineered to override satiety signals and light up reward circuits.

- **Speed and convenience.** Foods designed for autopilot, eaten without preparation or awareness.

- **Disorientation.** Confusing advice, misleading labels, and a deference to external authority that erodes trust in your body's signals.

At one level you're surrounded by foods engineered to be irresistible, effortless, and endless; at another level, you're within a system that makes conscious eating harder than ever. That's why you need practical defaults that bring back what's been taken away. These are the Five Power Moves, simple but foundational upgrades that rebuild a food environment where your Inner Eaters can shine.

POWER MOVE 1. EMPHASIZING REAL FOOD: RETURN TO EVOLUTIONARY ALIGNMENT

Here we are, spinning on a planet hurtling through space, watching our civilization simultaneously undermine the only biosphere we know while we scroll through food delivery apps and debate whether oat milk or almond milk is more sustainable. In the midst of this chaos, there's something profoundly grounding about returning to food that has nourished humans for millennia.

Michael Pollan nailed it with elegant simplicity: "Eat food. Not too much. Mostly plants."[1] He makes clear in his book that he means "real" food. Real food means food made with ingredients your ancestors would recognize, like vegetables, legumes, fruits, whole grains, nuts, seeds, and herbs raised in healthy soil, and animals raised eating those healthy ingredients.

The power move of *returning to evolutionary alignment* (REAL) does not mean eating like a paleolithic caveman (unless you're inclined to skin a wild rabbit with a stone tool for dinner). It does, however, mean recognizing that your body still runs on ancient biology, not the artificially sweetened, ultraprocessed rhythms of Food 2.0.

While opting for whole, unprocessed foods is generally a good move, remember that your biology is unique. The same "healthy" foods that energize your friend might trigger inflammation in your system. Genetics, microbiome, and lifestyle all shape how you respond to different foods. Some people thrive on high-fiber diets, while others experience bloating and digestive distress. Some people tolerate high-fat diets and maintain healthy blood lipids; others cannot.

Your body, your REAL rules. Become your own nutritional detective. Notice how different real foods affect your energy, digestion, and mood. Pair this with regular blood work to see how dietary shifts impact essential biomarkers like inflammation, liver enzymes, and glucose regulation.

The beauty of emphasizing real foods is that it creates a nutrient-dense foundation while allowing for personal customization. The point is not to eat 100 percent unprocessed foods— that would be untenable and impossible. You will eat ultraprocessed food. That is a fact. What matters is that the choice lies within you rather than the forces of Food 2.0.

When you return to evolutionary alignment, your:

- **Survival Eater** feels satisfied by nutrients it recognizes.

- **Pleasure Eater** enjoys the depth and flavor of real ingredients.

- **Social Eater** appreciates food made by human hands or grown locally.

- **Strategic Eater** plays the long game of health and vitality.

POWER MOVE 2. GOING SLOW:
SET LIMITS ON WARP-SPEED LIVING

Your stomach doesn't have WiFi. It can't text you when it needs attention or a well-deserved break. It operates on ancient rhythms that require your actual presence to perceive its signals, something increasingly rare in our hyperconnected world where every moment is colonized by productivity demands, information streams, and the relentless acceleration of what we politely call "modern life."

The power move of *setting limits on warp speed* living (SLOW) is the antidote to Food 2.0's speed and distraction. Food 2.0 keeps you eating while stressed, scrolling, and multitasking—calories that barely register as a meal. But our bodies evolved to function at the pace of seasons, sunrises, and the time it takes for an apple to ripen.

SLOW means:

- **Screen-free meals**. Creating phone-free zones so eating can take center stage.

- **Reclaiming mealtime**. Scheduling more than a three-minute gap between your meetings—give yourself real time to eat.

- **Observing hunger.** Pausing before eating to check your hunger, breathing, and your Inner Eaters' desires.

- **Adding pauses**. Set down your utensils, sip water, and recenter yourself in the eating experience.

This isn't about being a monk at dinner. It's about getting your mind back into your body and eating with all your senses. It's also about reclaiming your right to rest and nourish yourself, unencumbered by work or the need to be productive.

When you set limits on warp speed, your:

- **Survival Eater** settles down because slow meals also signal *"I'm safe."*

- **Pleasure Eater** savors flavor as it unfolds moment by moment.

- **Social Eater** broadens attention to reconnect with yourself, your space, and others.

- **Strategic Eater** celebrates improved digestion as digestive enzymes do their work.

POWER MOVE 3. RETURN HOME: HACK OBSTACLES IN MODERN ENVIRONMENTS

Many modern food environments are designed to work against moderation and balance. Returning home means reclaiming your terrain. You may not control the global food system, but you can control the six feet around your fridge. By shaping your environment, you reduce friction, conserve willpower, and make aligned choices easier.

The power move of hacking obstacles in modern environments (HOME) means to:

- **Develop label literacy.** Ignore front-package marketing. Read ingredients. Look up what you don't recognize, and apply the Food 2.0 test: *Is this engineered to be irresistible, effortless, and endless?*

- **Create islands of intention.** Make your values visible on counters, in lunch bags, and at your desk. Let REAL foods be the first thing your eyes land on.

- **Use smart convenience.** Harness modern supermarket conveniences for good: Leverage meal kits, frozen vegetables, prewashed greens, and precooked proteins. Just keep your standards sharp—Ignore health halos ("Made with real fruit") and see through emotional marketing terms like *all-natural* that have no legal definition.

- **Batch cook and meal plan.** Cook once, eat multiple times. Build a few reliable go-to meals that save time and reduce decision fatigue.

When you don't rise to your aspirations, you fall to the level of your environment. Design that environment so your values always have home-court advantage.

POWER MOVE 4. STRENGTHEN TIES: TOGETHERNESS, INTENTION, ECOLOGY, STORY

Food 2.0 severed our ties to land, labor, and each other, thriving on isolated consumers lost in contradictory opinions about what's best to eat. Eating 2.0 reconnects you to the larger web of relationships that make your meals possible. It reminds you that every meal is more than a transaction, a calorie count, or a commodity; it's a way of participating in the ongoing unfolding of life itself.

Strengthening TIES means:

- **Togetherness.** Sharing meals when possible; cook and eat with others.

- **Intention.** Treat dining spaces as sacred, food preparation as worthy of care, and gratitude a centerpiece of every meal.

- **Ecology.** Acknowledging your place in living systems; support ecoconscious companies and regenerative farming practices when you can.

- **Story.** Let meals carry meaning beyond their nutrients by connecting with cultural food traditions. Invite friends to share food memories. Let your meals tell stories.

These TIES aren't luxury add-ons for those with time and money to spare. You don't need to buy your food directly from a farmer or cook every meal from scratch in order to remember that you are part of a much larger story, one that spans soil, hands, history, and hope. Even small moments of connection—thanking the cashier at the supermarket, considering the chicken who laid your egg, or sharing a simple meal with a coworker—help rewire your relationship with food and support eating as an infinite game best played with others.

POWER MOVE 5. FLEXIBLE CONSISTENCY: STRUCTURE THAT MOVES WITH YOU

Flexible consistency is a keystone habit for Eating 2.0—reinforcing your ability to maintain the preceding power moves without becoming brittle. It's choreography that helps you move with your day instead of getting knocked around by it. Think of it as the art of maintaining *accountability with elasticity*, honoring your commitment to your Inner Eaters while adapting to today's reality.

The key question to ask when life gets messy is: *Am I slipping into old habits, or am I evolving?* The answer lies in whether you can return to conscious leadership, not because you have to, but because it helps you feel like yourself again. Success isn't binary: you win or you fail. Success is returning to alignment.

Each time you stay in integrity with these power moves, you signal to your Inner Eaters that their needs matter, that you're

THE FIVE POWER MOVES OF EATING 2.0		
Power Move	**What It Adds Back**	**Tools/Habits**
Emphasize REAL	Whole nutrients and evolutionary alignment	Label literacy, Food 2.0 quick-test, macro-nutrient aware-ness, and market-ing discernment
Go SLOW	Satiety and presence	Screen-free meals, breathing pauses, fullness check-ins
Return HOME	Supportive food environment	Pantry/fridge audit, counter visibility, menu discernment, intentional shop-ping, and meal prep
Strengthen TIES	Connection and meaning	Family meals, local foods, traditional recipes, and cultural rituals
Flexible consistency	Integrity and trust	Reflect, reorient, refine and return. Adapt without losing alignment.

listening, and that you're committed to leading them toward sustainable nourishment rather than reactive consumption.

Your Systems Inventory

Building outer leadership starts with honest reflection about what's already working and what needs adjustment. So, before moving forward, take a moment to assess where you are in terms of the power moves described previously. Use these questions not to prove you're doing it "right," but to stay connected to what matters most.

Grab a pen and paper and write down your answers to the questions below.

REAL FOOD ASSESSMENT

What meals do you regularly eat that already feel good and align with your values?

Where could you add more whole, unprocessed foods without overwhelming yourself?

Which real foods make you feel most energized and satisfied, helping you play the long game of vitality and integrity?

SLOW LIVING CHECK-IN

How often do you eat while distracted or rushing?

Where's your biggest opportunity to slow down: breakfast, lunch, dinner, or snacks?

What would you need to change to make eating slower actually possible?

HOME ENVIRONMENT AUDIT

Where do you most often default to reactive food choices? What's one simple change you could make to your kitchen, meal routine, or grocery habits to help you make smart choices easier?

Which "island of intention" could you create without massive amounts of work—your counter, desk, or lunch bag?

TIES REFLECTION

How could you use food experiences to strengthen your connections with people, places, and traditions?

What food stories or mealtime memories matter to you?

Where might you support food systems that align with your values?

FLEXIBLE CONSISTENCY

When your plans are thrown off, how can you remember your shared vision and empower your Inner Eaters toward that vision?

What does "bending without breaking" look like for you when dining out or grocery shopping?

When you slip into old eating habits, how will you get back to conscious leadership?

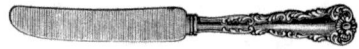

YOU DON'T NEED to tackle everything at once. Start by noticing where your current structure supports you and where it works against you. Even small adjustments in your outer environment can create significant shifts in how your Inner Eaters show up. And remember, there's no final win or perfect setup, only your evolving leadership in the face of Food 2.0 reality.

Looking Ahead:
Leading Through the Mess

Even the best-designed systems break down. You'll forget to go grocery shopping. A work deadline will derail your ability to go slow. You'll find yourself sitting on the couch with a drink in hand even if you said you wanted to break that habit loop.

Life is messy, and in the next chapter, we'll explore how to lead your Inner Eaters when both your inner leadership and outer systems fall apart.

ELEVEN

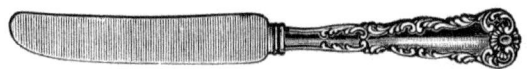

MAKING PEACE WITH FOOD
HARMONIZING THE DESIRES THAT PULL YOU APART

"Systems are perfectly designed to achieve the results they are currently achieving. In other words, no matter how dysfunctional a system appears to be, it is producing benefits for the people who participate in it."

DAVID PETER STROH

Casey's week with food told a familiar story of being pulled in different directions. On Sunday, she walked into the grocery store with a neat list in hand. By the time she reached the checkout, the cart told a different tale: a frozen pizza her daughter begged for, a box of protein bars that caught her eye, and a family-size bag of chips on sale.

Casey didn't feel guilty; she was just confused about how her clear intentions at the start had blurred once she was in the store.

The next morning, a coworker passed around a basket of warm donuts. Casey's Pleasure Eater perked up: "*Nothing beats fresh* donuts." Her Strategic Eater frowned: "*If you eat this now, you won't be hungry for lunch later.*" Her Social Eater added: "*Take one, or you'll look uptight.*" Casey tore off a piece while joining the small talk, but halfway through, she realized she hadn't tasted it at all—just eaten while negotiating with herself.

That evening, she slumped onto the couch, phone in hand, scrolling through delivery apps. Burgers, burritos, sushi, salads—the choices faded together. Her Pleasure Eater lobbied for the burger she'd seen in an ad earlier. Her Strategic Eater whispered that she really should cook something from the fridge. Ten minutes later, she was still scrolling. Nothing had been ordered.

Casey was tired of feeling like food decisions were tiny negotiations she never fully won. When your Inner Eaters pull in different directions, even normal eating moments can feel incredibly draining.

This is where examining your eating challenges matters: Not to pathologize normal behaviors or create more rules, but to identify where simple systems might lighten your mental load and help you make peace with food.

Get Honest about Your Eating Challenges

Casey's week isn't unusual. It's a mirror of the quiet negotiations most of us face. The details may change, but the pattern is the same: clear intentions slipping, inner voices clashing, and energy drained by the back-and-forth. The first move toward making peace with food is honesty—naming what's truly happening in your relationship with food instead of pretending it's fine.

Like family members who've been living together for years, your Inner Eaters have established patterns of interacting with each other: alliances, rivalries, and coping strategies that may have once helped but now create more problems than they solve. Conscious leadership begins by getting honest with yourself about what's really going on.

Where does your eating feel most off track?

Have you been breaking promises to yourself? If so, what were they?

And here's a big consideration: Is today's struggle part of a pattern you keep running into?

If this line of inquiry feels overwhelming, threatening, or just irrelevant to you, that's totally fine. Let's not make problems where there are none. As I said in previous chapters, you are not wrong, lesser, broken, or in any way unworthy for eating the way you currently do.

The content of this chapter runs the risk of turning normal eating into a project requiring constant self-monitoring that creates more stress, not less. That is not the intention. If you have eating challenges that make you feel out of sorts and wanting something new, give these tools a try. If not, I suggesting reading along to build your awareness anyway. There's always room for improvement.

SPOT THE PATTERNS:
SOFTEN THE SHADOW

When your Inner Eaters operate from fear or past pain, they display characteristic shadow patterns that can hijack your entire eating experience. Unfortunately, you can't just demand that your Inner Eaters get back in line. It's like dealing with an upset kid, you have to help them calm down first, then figure out how to play nicely with the others.

Here's a quick reference guide to recognize each Inner Eater's shadow. You can also find more extensive descriptions in Part Two.

The **Survival Eater's shadow** involves:

- Impulsive eating driven by urgent now-or-never energy.
- Opportunistic consumption—eating simply because food is available.
- Difficulty stopping even when physically satisfied.
- Persistent anxiety about having "enough," regardless of actual abundance.

Warning signs to watch out for include hoarding food, grazing absentmindedly, and eating whatever portions are offered regardless of hunger.

The **Pleasure Eater's shadow** involves:

- Hedonistic patterns where taste trumps all other considerations.
- Insatiable cravings where one indulgence leads immediately to another.
- Extreme pickiness or food rejection.
- Emotional numbing through pleasure foods and overeating.

Warning signs to watch out for include obsessing over particular foods, rejecting perfectly good foods, chasing novelty over nourishment, and endlessly seeking more.

The **Social Eater's shadow** involves:

- People-pleasing behaviors where you consistently override your own needs to match social expectations.
- Contrarian patterns where you reflexively oppose group norms to assert independence, or judging others' eating as a way to feel superior.

- Turning meals into social media content or choosing foods primarily for how they'll appear to others.

- Feeling intense embarrassment about your food preferences, cultural eating practices, or family food traditions.

Warning signs to look out for include eating to fit in (even when it causes harm), or eating defiantly to prove a point rather than from genuine preference.

The **Strategic Eater's shadow** involves:

- Rigid all-or-nothing thinking where unplanned food choices feel like complete failure.

- Creating elaborate rationales for food choices after the fact, rather than making decisions based on actual needs in the moment.

- Attachment to dietary dogma, experts, or influencers that override your bodily wisdom.

- Excessive focus on metrics (calories, macros) at the expense of actual experience.

Warning signs to look out for include obsessing over "perfect" plans, falling into black-and-white thinking, and giving up and checking out (*What the hell, I blew it*).

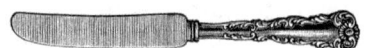

ONCE YOU'VE IDENTIFIED which Inner Eater is operating from its shadow, approach it with curiosity rather than criticism. It's worth remembering that even when your Inner Eaters are acting like complete jerks, they're usually trying to protect something that matters.

Ask the imbalanced part: *What are you trying to protect? What do you need right now that you're not getting?* Listen for the deeper need beneath the reactive behavior. This is about understanding its purpose so you can help this part of you express its gifts rather than its fears.

From Conflict to Collaboration: Six Strategies for Working with Your Whole System

Once you've addressed the obvious shadow patterns of individual Inner Eaters, it's time to work with your whole internal system. This takes everything you've learned about leadership, plus some new skills for handling serious disagreements and complete system breakdowns.

Please remember, however, that none of this is a formulaic fix. These strategies are part of an ongoing practice of conscious leadership, which is strengthened through experience, careful experimentation, and sometimes, with professional support.

Here are six strategies for getting your Inner Eater back on the same team with one another.

STRATEGY 1. MAP AND TRANSFORM YOUR POWER DYNAMICS

Before you can lead your eating system, you need to see who has habitually been taking the steering wheel. You might have established patterns of dominance that no longer serve you.

You can put it into practice by:

- **Drawing a relationship map.** Create a simple diagram showing which Inner Eaters currently dominate your food decisions.

- **Identifying silenced voices.** Which Inner Eaters are consistently ignored or overruled?

- **Naming specific alliances.** For example, *My Social Eater often sides with my Strategic Eater against my Pleasure Eater.*

- **Exploring with compassion.** *What is this alliance trying to protect me from? What fear drives this pattern?*

The purpose of mapping your power dynamics is to help create clear boundaries, because when roles overlap or when everyone tries to be the decision-maker, confusion emerges and nothing gets done well. No single Inner Eater should manage the others.

STRATEGY 2. THE "GOOD ENOUGH" APPROACH

Perfect solutions that fully satisfy every Inner Eater rarely exist. That's okay. Instead, aim for "good enough" choices that keep everyone engaged in the ongoing conversation.

Think of it like planning a road trip with friends who have different skills—one person navigates, another handles music, someone else manages snacks, and another watches the budget. Nobody tries to do everything, but everyone contributes what they do best.

You can put it into practice by:

- **Checking with your Survival Eater first.** *What does my body actually need right now?*

- **Consulting your Pleasure Eater about the experience.** *What would make this meal satisfying and enjoyable?*

- **Asking your Social Eater about the context**. *How can I honor the social aspect of this meal?*

- **Getting input from your Strategic Eater on alignment**. *How does this align with my values?*

The magic isn't in finding perfection—it's in weaving these voices into a workable decision you can live with.

STRATEGY 3. TAKING TURNS IN THE SPOTLIGHT

Sometimes, wise leadership means letting one Inner Eater lead on purpose. Your Strategic Eater might lead before a workout; your Pleasure Eater might take over at a celebration. This isn't a problem unless the same Inner Eater dominates every meal all of the time without conscious choice. This would be like letting your oldest child always pick the family movie. Eventually, the others revolt.

You can put it into practice by:

- **Creating guardrails.** For instance, allowing an Inner Eater to take the spotlight twice in a row, but not three times.

- **Cheerleading.** When a part gets the limelight, truly let it shine. Be its cheerleader. Empower it to find its healthiest expression.

- **Handling pushback.** Reassure your other Inner Eaters they're not forgotten. Say: *I hear your concern, and I'm choosing a different path based on this particular context.*

- **Debriefing.** *How did that feel? How did it affect the whole Inner Eater family system? What might restore balance to the next meal?*

This strategy works best when you let each Inner Eater do what they do best. When your Survival Eater tries to make social decisions or your Social Eater attempts to calculate nutrition, you get suboptimal results. But when each one stays in their lane and contributes their unique strengths, the whole system functions more effectively.

STRATEGY 4. DECIDE FROM TOMORROW, FOR TODAY

When cravings clash with values, borrow wisdom from your future self. Ask: *What would tomorrow-me thank me for today?*

Sometimes the answer is a salad. Sometimes it's the ice cream and joy that came with it. The key is answering the question from holistic perspective of conscious leadership, not from a single Inner Eater's urgency. It's not *either* "right now" *or* "tomorrow." It is *"both . . . and . . . ."*

This approach works especially well when you tend toward immediate gratification. It adds a layer of space and grace to not take things so seriously. Imagine what "future you" might tell you *not to worry about.*

Getting into the mindset of your future self enables you to let go of little things (even if they seem like big things in the moment) because weeks, months, and years from now, they probably aren't as significant as they seem.

STRATEGY 5. FINDING SHARED HOPE

Beneath the bickering, every Inner Eater hopes for a better future: Your job is to find that hope, look for shared ground, and remind them when they forget.

You can put it into practice by:

- **Exploring what each Inner Eater genuinely hopes for.** For instance, your Strategic Eater might hope for alignment between choices and values, and your Pleasure Eater might hope for more joy and spontaneity.

- **Affirming your capacity to begin again.** *We can do this. There's a way forward*—this matters more than getting it right the first time.

- **Crafting a compelling narrative.** Tell a story where the future is worth striving for—dream big.

- **Celebrating even small steps toward that shared vision.**

Hope reframes struggle as purposeful. It keeps you moving forward when the process gets messy.

STRATEGY 6. LETTING IT BE MESSY

Here's a counterintuitive truth: Sometimes the wisest move is no move at all. Don't rush to fix the discomfort; rather, skillfully make space for it.

What I've discovered is that some of our greatest suffering around food comes from our intolerance of discomfort and our rush to fix it. Our culture tells us that we can buy our way out of any bad feeling, but what if emotional tension—wanting many things but only getting one—is part of being a healthy human? This dynamic push-pull is what makes our eating come alive, and there are times we need to let the discomfort breathe.

When your Inner Eaters are in heated debate, instead of imposing agreement, try taking the following steps.

1. Pause. Don't rush to resolve your discomfort.

2. Do your best to transcend the action, the feelings, and the stories, as if you are stepping onto a balcony and looking down at them from above.

3. Observe any tension you feel as energy in your body, nothing more.

4. Let your Inner Eaters argue—it's part of the process.

5. Notice how the energy eventually changes.

Our culture gravitates towards quick fixes—one pill for every ill. It's hard to shift this mindset because we've become allergic to even the slightest discomfort. But sitting in the awkwardness of feeling a multitude of emotions and not knowing what happens next is precisely what allows new possibilities to emerge. Your next best move may appear, not from forcing harmony, but from allowing creative tension to do its work.

Making Invisible Conversations Visible

One of the most powerful techniques for evolving your Inner Eater relationships is facilitating direct conversations between them. Though it might feel unfamiliar at first, this practice can be incredibly healing.

Imagine you're standing in the kitchen, and part of you wants the pint of salted caramel gelato. Another part says, "*Just call it a night.*" A third part whispers, "*You promised your partner you'd eat healthier.*" These back-and-forth debates are proof that you're human.

Instead of letting your Pleasure Eater, Strategic Eater, and Social Eater battle it out, what if you helped them talk it through?

Here's a sequence of steps with which to practice constructive dialogues.

1. **Name what you're feeling.** Get quiet and focus on the feelings inside your body. Try to name them with as much clarity as possible.

2. **Name what you're hearing.** What are the stories running through your head? Can you identify and describe the narratives?

3. **Identify the Inner Eaters.** How are these thoughts and feelings linked with your Inner Eaters? Can you distinguish their voices? Can you discern their concern?

4. **Ask each perspective one question**, such as:

   - *"Strategic Eater, why do you feel threatened by dessert?"*

   - *"Pleasure Eater, what do you wish Strategic Eater understood about your needs?"*

   - *"Social Eater, how do you feel when Survival Eater makes impulsive choices without considering other people?"*

5. **Listen with genuine openness**: Let part of you speak fully before inviting the others to respond. Encourage each Inner Eater to express its feelings, needs, and concerns as clearly as possible. You're not forcing agreement; you're creating space for understanding.

At first, this dialogue practice might feel silly. You might wonder: *Am I really having conversations with parts of myself?* This hesitation is completely normal.

If it makes you feel less cuckoo when you're having the conversation, remember that you're not fragmenting your identity; you're recognizing the natural complexity that exists within you (and all the rest of us, too). This approach draws on established therapeutic traditions that understand how internal dialogue can resolve conflicts that keep us stuck in unhelpful patterns.

With practice, these invisible conversations become more fluid and natural. You'll spend less time trapped in food confusion and more time experiencing the integrated wisdom that emerges when all aspects of yourself are welcomed to the table.

CASEY'S COUNCIL TABLE:
A RESOLUTION STORY

Months later, Casey's week looked different. The grocery store still tempted her with sales and snacks, but now she paused at the cart, mapping her Inner Eaters' voices before heading to checkout. Her Pleasure Eater could still ask for chips, but her Strategic and Survival Eaters got a say too, making sure fruits, proteins, and easy staples were in place. It wasn't about perfect control, but about power dynamics: each part of her system had a chance to chime in.

At work, when the donuts came around, Casey practiced the "good enough" approach. Instead of getting stuck in debate, she let each Inner Eater weigh in, and then cut a donut in half, savoring the flavor with her Pleasure Eater while reassuring her Strategic side that this choice still fit the bigger picture.

At night, scrolling through delivery apps, Casey caught herself in the familiar loop. Instead of spiraling, she used "decide from tomorrow, for today." *What would future me thank me for?* Sometimes that meant keeping it easy and ordering out, other times it meant pulling together a simple meal from her fridge. Either way, she trusted the decision because it came from leadership, not autopilot.

At her nephew's birthday, Casey used to tense up when dessert appeared. This time, she tapped into shared hope: All her Inner Eaters wanted a future where food can mark a milestone in the life of someone she cared about. So, she ate the cake, laughing with her family and recognizing that moments like this were rare.

Casey's Inner Eaters had become advisors, not dictators. For the first time, she was able to create "good enough" balance, meal by meal, in a way that felt sustainable.

Casey was embodying many of the principles of Eating 2.0, making food choices an integrated expression of her whole self. Curiosity opened her awareness. Appreciation softened the shadows of her extreme parts. She took responsibility for the internal power dynamics, allowing her to truly lead. Lastly, she explored how to make eating decisions that felt both smart and sensible, without resorting to old habits that kept her unhappy.

When Your Eating Goes Off Track: Restoring Dynamic Harmony

Even with the best intentions and tools, your relationship with food will sometimes feel out of balance. Maybe it's a single event— a late-night binge, an emotional eating episode, or an unexpected crisis that launches you into impulsive eating. Or perhaps it's a gradual drift: mindless snacking during Netflix marathons, vacation indulgences, or a season where food takes a backseat to other priorities.

As the quote at the beginning of the chapter says, systems are perfectly designed to achieve the results they're currently achieving—even if it's dysfunctional. That familiar way of eating might be the very imbalance you're trying to transform.

The first step? Release the pressure to "do it right." You need to compare the benefits of change with the benefits of maintaining the status quo. Change always entails risk, and you inevitably will lose some comforting habits along the way. You have to believe that the payoffs of eating differently will be better than what you're getting now.

Return to the core values you mapped out in Chapter 4 and start to let go of current ways of eating that do not serve these higher aspirations. Reread the chapters on each Inner Eater to get to know this part of yourself better. Then work with your Inner Eaters, both individually and collectively, to compassionately reprogram their patterns to align around what is most important for you.

As the conscious leader, you will have to make hard decisions. You will have to take responsibility for your actions. You will also need to anticipate the bumps in the road ahead: the moments when you feel like nothing is working, and you're entering the territory of shame. Food 2.0 will tempt you to resort to old, unconscious eating habits. The best way forward is to move slowly, gently, at the speed of trust. If you don't trust your Inner Eaters, they'll have no reason to trust you. Once trust is in place, you can upgrade your eating operating system without falling into the subtle violence of self-improvement or the inertia of the status quo.

KNOW WHEN TO ASK FOR HELP

These practices can help with the stress that comes with navigating modern food environments. But some situations benefit from professional support, and there's wisdom in recognizing when you need more help than self-leadership alone can provide. If you're experiencing significant distress around eating, reaching out to a qualified therapist, dietitian, or coach who understands disordered eating can provide the external perspective and support needed for deeper healing.

Consider reaching out to a qualified professional if:

- Your eating patterns are significantly impacting your physical health, relationships, or daily functioning.

- You have a history of disordered eating and notice familiar patterns returning.

- You're using food to cope with trauma, depression, or anxiety in ways that concern you.

- The Inner Eater framework has revealed longstanding patterns, and you need more intensive support to work through these eating challenges.

The Inner Eater framework can be used in conjunction with therapy, nutrition counseling, or medical care, but it's not a substitute for professional help. I know it can be tempting to think you don't need others; you can do it all on your own. I was this way for years, perhaps decades. But I've come to understand that asking for help isn't weakness; it's wisdom. None of us was meant to navigate the journey to upgraded eating alone.

Taking Your Eating 2.0 Operating System Live

Now that you've built the capacity to lead your Inner Eaters through disagreement and disconnection, let's bring this leadership into the wider world. In the next chapter, we'll explore how to navigate social eating situations while maintaining dynamic harmony, inner leadership, and outer mastery.

Ultimately, the real test of your Eating 2.0 operating system won't be how well you do in controlled environments, but how skillfully you can navigate the complex, unpredictable world of eating well with others in an era of superabundance.

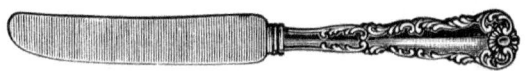

TWELVE

EATING 2.0 IN THE REAL WORLD
NAVIGATING RESTAURANTS, SUPERMARKETS, AND SOCIAL TABLES

"The Church says: The body is a sin.
Science says: The body is a machine.
Advertising says: The body is a business.
The Body says: I am a fiesta."

EDUARDO GALEANO

Airports. Office parties. Family dinners. The late-night kitchen raid. This is where the rubber meets the road—where your Inner Eaters don't care what you've read, only what you choose to eat.

This chapter is your field manual for navigating ten common scenarios where normal food decision-making turns into everyday eating struggles. Here's your chance to bring Eating 2.0 into the real world to feed your real life.

Grounding Principles for Eating 2.0

Before diving into specific situations, let's resurface the key principles that will serve as your decision anchors for your Eating 2.0 operating system.

Lead with CARE, not control. Controlling food decisions through rigidity, willpower, or fear only reinforces internal conflict. Instead, approach each eating situation with curiosity, appreciation, responsibility, and exploration.

Make conscious tradeoffs, not perfect choices. Food 2.0 is engineered to be irresistible, endless, and effortless. You will eat it— and that's fine. The goal isn't to eliminate Food 2.0 from your life but to become the type of eater who can navigate this landscape without feeling overwhelmed or disempowered. Every choice has tradeoffs. Aim to choose with clarity rather than sleepwalking through your hunger.

Design your defaults. The system is stacked against you, optimized for speed, shelf life, and profit, not your well-being. You can't control the broader food environment, but you can shape your immediate environment: your fridge, your pantry, your shopping list, and your counter.

Messy is normal. Conflict between your Inner Eaters isn't a sign something's wrong; it's evidence you're navigating a complex food environment. Disagreement can energize your eating system when handled skillfully. Make space for learning to occur.

Practice until it's natural. Integration isn't one breakthrough moment. It's something you practice repeatedly through lived experience. When things feel tangled, return to your systematic tools: Map the dynamics, find "good enough" solutions, take turns in the spotlight, decide from tomorrow, reconnect to shared hope, repeat.

Learning to Lead:
The Progression

Like any complex skill—from learning to drive to developing emotional intelligence—mastering your Inner Eater leadership unfolds through predictable stages that cannot be rushed. Understanding this natural progression helps you meet yourself with patience and realistic expectations as these new capacities develop.

STAGE 1. RETROSPECTIVE AWARENESS: THE LOOKING BACK STAGE

Most people start their Eating 2.0 journey with retrospective awareness, reflecting on their eating only after the plate is clean, the bag is empty, or the meal is over. This is completely normal and necessary. You can look back on any eating experience and learn from it. The key is skillful reflection. Ask:

- *What just happened?*
- *Who (which Inner Eater) was in charge?*
- *What was I prioritizing? Was that a choice or a default?*
- *What information does this give me for next time?*

This stage can last weeks, months, or years. Like learning to recognize your own patterns in relationships or work, developing self-awareness around eating takes time. Don't rush the development of this foundation. Every meal you consider more in depth is a move towards more conscious eating.

STAGE 2. ANTICIPATORY AWARENESS:
THE SEEING IT COMING STAGE

With consistent practice, reflection becomes anticipation. You begin to notice tensions before meals—the stress building, the hunger ignored for too long, the social pressure mounting. You also begin to deliberately think about how your Inner Eaters will behave in upcoming eating situations. For instance, if you're planning a big dinner out, you start imagining your Social Eater discussing the menu or your Survival Eater growing hungry with anticipation.

This stage looks like:

- Recognizing triggers before they fully activate. *I'm getting that scattered feeling that usually leads to stress eating*

- Anticipating Inner Eater conflicts. *My Strategic Eater is about to clash with my Pleasure Eater at this restaurant.*

- Planning for challenging situations. *Family dinners always turn my Social Eater into an appeaser—how can I prepare?*

The key skills are thinking ahead with Storytelling Vision to see you are bigger than any of these default reactions. Then, using the Inner Eater framework, proactively map out your eating experience, so you can enter into your next meal with as much awareness and appreciation as possible. All this forethought is helpful, but no matter how much you plan ahead, you can never fully predict what will happen in the moment—embrace the uncertainty and stay adaptive—the conscious leader doesn't cling to one way.

STAGE 3. REAL-TIME AWARENESS:
THE WHILE EATING STAGE

This is where you begin noticing Inner Eater dynamics while they're occurring during an eating experience. You catch yourself mid-bite, pause during meals, and facilitate real-time collaboration between your Inner Eaters.

In this stage, you're noticing and making conscious course corrections as you eat. For example, you might observe *I'm eating fast because my Survival Eater is anxious—let me slow down.*

Stage 3 requires significant neural rewiring to stay connected to your experience as it unfolds. Like learning to stay present during difficult conversations instead of getting hijacked by strong emotions, this capacity develops gradually through consistent practice. Expect this to be inconsistent at first—some meals you'll have it, others you won't.

At this stage, it can be helpful to rely heavily on the structures and frameworks in this book. You're still learning how to work with your Inner Eaters, and this requires scaffolding and focus. However, there is a danger of thinking you understand or have more control than you do. You must be aware of when assumptions are failing, when interactions are shifting, or when one part is being triggered. Over time, you'll begin to internalize the Inner Eater framework, recognize those moments (for example, stress, travel, fatigue) that act as tipping points where your internal system easily flips into old patterns. Rather than collapsing, you'll be ready to respond using the CARE process and all the harmonization strategies you've learned thus far. But first, you need deliberate practice and a willingness for it to be messy.

STAGE 4. EMBODIED EATING 2.0: THE INTEGRATION STAGE

In this mature stage, Eating 2.0 becomes increasingly natural and effortless. You don't have to rely so much on the Inner Eater framework as this way of thinking and operating have become integrated into your way of being. Eating at this stage becomes a fluid dance of awareness, choice, and adaptation.

In Stage 4, you can expect:

- Eating consciously to feel natural and unforced, like breathing.

- Inner Eater disagreement as healthy and helpful perspectives to consider.

- To adapt fluidly to different situations without losing your capacity to lead.

- Food to be whatever you want it to be—nourishment, pleasure, connection, achievement—without you needing it to be any of these things.

This stage represents unconscious competence with conscious availability. Like an experienced driver who doesn't think about every gear shift but can instantly respond to unexpected situations, you eat naturally while maintaining the ability to bring conscious attention to your parts when needed.

This stage can take years to fully develop, and you may move in and out of it depending on how many major changes or new challenges you're facing.

Keep in mind that some people move through stages quickly, others more slowly. Factors like stress levels, support systems, past trauma, and natural temperament all influence your development. Don't compare yourself with others—it's counterproductive. This is your eating journey. Move at your own pace.

THE PROGRESSION

Retrospective Awareness → Anticipatory Awareness →
Real-time Awareness → Embodied Eating 2.0.

Ten Real-World Scenarios

Now, let's take this framework into ten real-world scenarios where Eating 2.0 gets tested, and where your Inner Eater leadership skills can truly shine.

SCENARIO 1. WORK EVENTS, SOCIAL GATHERINGS, AND SPECIAL OCCASIONS

It starts with the champagne. You didn't plan to drink tonight; this was just a networking mixer. But now someone's handed you a flute, smiling, watching. You're standing next to the VP you admire. Trays of hors d'oeuvres drift past like clockwork.

Your Social Eater does not want to look awkward. It wants to fit in. Your Strategic Eater is wondering if this is going to be one of the "f— it" nights. The old operating system kicks in.

Option 1. Eat everything in sight and hate yourself later.

Option 2. White-knuckle your way through the night, declining delicious food with awkward apologies.

Both options are stuck in single perspectives. Neither feels good because they're missing the larger picture.

The Eating 2.0 shift. You don't need to leave the event, but you can adopt a new mindset. Get curious about the voices inside you. Appreciate that your Social Eater craves connection and your Strategic

Eater values integrity—both valid needs. Take responsibility for making conscious choices rather than reacting impulsively.

CONSCIOUS LEADERSHIP STRATEGIES

BEFORE THE EVENT:

- **Set an intention.** Shift the focus from food as a problem to food as part of the larger experience you want to create—connection, joy, ease, celebration.
- **Eat normally.** Don't arrive starving or overly restricted.
- **Remember the real nourishment.** When the buffet overwhelms you, or when social anxiety spikes, pause and remember your intention. Put your energy and attention on the thing you came for.

DURING THE GATHERING:

- **Survey before choosing.** What foods stand out or are truly special? What foods are items you buy or make at home?
- **Create distance from constant temptation.** Don't camp next to the appetizer table or bar.
- **Pause before each choice to reflect.** *What part of me is choosing this?*
- **Seek connection beyond consumption.** Focus your energy on conversations, stories, and relationships.

AFTER THE EVENT:

- **Appreciate the experience.** Both the food and the connection it facilitated.

- **Reflect without judgment.** What did you enjoy eating? What could you have passed up? What would make the next event even more satisfying?

- **Return to what serves you.** Tomorrow isn't about "making up for" tonight—it's about returning to what makes you feel like yourself.

SCENARIO 2. FAMILY MEALS WITH FOOD PUSHERS

You've already eaten plenty of food, but here comes your aunt, beaming, insistent, holding a second helping of lasagna like a gift. "Come on, sweetheart. You used to love this. Just one more piece."

Your stomach tightens, not from hunger, but from expectation.

Your Social Eater wants to keep the peace. Your Strategic Eater screams, *"No, you're already full."* Your Pleasure Eater feels confused. You used to love this dish, but now it's tangled in pressure and resentment.

The old script kicks in.

Option 1. Say yes with a fake smile, eat past fullness, and feel bitter.

Option 2. Say no defensively, create distance, and make the room feel colder.

Either way, food wins and connection suffers.

The Eating 2.0 Shift. You don't need to prove anything, not your loyalty, not your self-control. Get curious about what's really happening: this food offering is about love, culture, and nostalgia. Appreciate the care behind the offer while respecting your body's signals.

You can honor the meaning behind this food—connection to family and tradition—without eating more than feels good in your body. It is not all or nothing. It just takes some courage, a tactful tone, and a willingness to rock the boat (if need be).

CONSCIOUS LEADERSHIP STRATEGIES

BEFORE THE GATHERING:

- **Understand the family system.** What role does food play? How can you connect without compromising yourself?

- **Rehearse kind responses.** Try "This looks amazing! Can I take some home for later?" or "I just finished my meal, but I'd love the recipe."

- **Define your boundaries.** What's nonnegotiable and where are you willing to flex?

DURING FAMILY INTERACTIONS:

- **Make eye contact and smile warmly.** Let them know you see the care behind the offer.

- **Redirect with appreciation.** "Your cooking is incredible! Can I just try a taste?" or "I'm saving room for dessert."

- **Find an alternative connection.** Such as "Tell me more about your recent trip" or "I remember when you first made this. Do you remember . . . ?"

- **Practice flexible consistency.** Your boundary might look different at Thanksgiving than on Tuesday night. Don't lose sight of the broader context.

FOR LONG-TERM FAMILY DYNAMICS:

- **Expect gradual change.** Family patterns shift slowly. If it feels impossible to say no, figure out what kind of supports would get you closer to holding your boundary next time.

- **Find allies.** Look for relatives who respect your boundaries and can model different interactions.

- **Honor thyself.** You can respect family food traditions, but ultimately, boundaries are not agreements—they're what you need to safely interact with the world.

SCENARIO 3. LATE-NIGHT EATING

It's 10:17 PM. The dishes are done, work emails are off, and you're finally ready to unwind. You've been running on adrenaline all day, meeting everyone else's expectations.

You don't remember walking to the kitchen, but there you are, leaning against the counter, holding a spoon, eyeing the ice cream.

Your Survival Eater kicks in: *"Just a little. Don't go to bed hungry."* Your Pleasure Eater joins: *"We didn't get any joy today. This is it."*

Remember that Food 2.0 doesn't just sell calories; it sells relief. It whispers: *"You earned this."* Before you know it, you've gone from "just a bite" to finishing the entire pint, not because you're weak, but because you're *spent*. Food 2.0 is designed to find you there with a spoon in hand.

The Eating 2.0 Shift. Get curious about what's driving this late-night eating. Appreciate that your Inner Eaters are trying to care for something important—rest, joy, comfort after a hard day. Take responsibility for pausing the autopilot. Explore options that honor your Inner Eaters' gifts, not their wounds.

CONSCIOUS LEADERSHIP STRATEGIES

BEFORE THE EVENING:

- **Review your day.** Were meals substantial and satisfying? Have you been eating real food or engineered snacks?

- **Create power-down routines.** Plan ahead to include things such as music, journaling, a shower, or whatever else signals the shift from work to rest.

- **Honor your nervous system's need to decompress.** Anticipate the need to "check out" without immediately reaching for food as the release valve.

DURING THE NIGHT HUNGER:

- **Pause and breathe.** Step away from the kitchen, sit down, and place a hand on your belly. Inhale deeply. Meet your hunger as energy in your body.

- **Get curious and reflect.** *What part of me is reaching for food? Survival, Pleasure, Social, or Strategic?*

- **If truly hungry, honor it with real food.** Choose to eat something that future you would be proud of rather than "sneaking" processed options.

- **Appreciate the complexity of being human.** *I'm eating because I'm tired/stressed/ lonely, and that's okay.*

FOR ONGOING INTEGRATION:

- **Notice patterns.** Does late-night eating follow certain triggers or circumstances? Does it happen at a certain time?

- **Examine your dinner satisfaction.** What truly satisfies versus what leaves you wanting more later?

- **Explore your eating rhythm.** Consider whether meals throughout the day need modification. Have you eaten enough?

- **Practice flexible consistency.** Some nights, chocolate at 10 PM feels great; other nights, it's emotional numbing. Your job is to figure out when you're acting from awareness and when you're on autopilot.

SCENARIO 4. AIRPORTS, TRAVEL, AND CONVENIENCE EATING

You're already feeling anxious about your long flight. Security took forever and you skipped breakfast. Your plane boards in thirty-eight minutes, and you're power-walking past overpriced food courts, scanning options like a tactical mission.

Pizza. Pretzels. Burgers. The smell of cinnamon sugar hits you. Your stomach growls. Your Pleasure Eater starts bargaining.

Your Survival Eater screams: *"Let's eat something now. There are all these options."* Your Strategic Eater counters: *"I don't see any wholesome choices."* Your Pleasure Eater chimes in: *"We're traveling. Smell that fresh-baked cinnamon roll—that would be delicious."*

Meanwhile, your blood sugar drops, patience evaporates, and the old unconscious operating system kicks in.

The Eating 2.0 Shift. Get curious about what you're actually facing: Airports are a decision fatigue battlefield designed to profit from your depletion. Appreciate that your Inner Eaters are responding to real constraints and disrupted routines. Take responsibility for leading within the system you're in, not the one you wish you had.

CONSCIOUS LEADERSHIP STRATEGIES

BEFORE DEPARTING:

- **Anchor with consistency.** Start your travel day with one familiar meal that satisfies all your Inner Eaters as best as you can.

- **Pack strategic snacks.** Give your Strategic Eater bargaining chips with real, nourishing options.

- **Research destinations.** Identify opportunities to be proactive in your food choices rather than reactive.

- **Set realistic expectations.** You're learning how to travel and nourish yourself well. Don't expect perfection or just give up and eat without any intention.

WHILE TRAVELING:

- **Pause to scan options.** Even under time pressure, ask, *Is this irresistible, effortless, and endless?* This is about conscious choice, not restrictive control.

- **Stay hydrated.** Thirst often masquerades as hunger and long periods of sitting can dehydrate you.

- **Practice balance.** "I'll try the local specialty *and* include vegetables when possible."

- **Use disruption as data.** Notice how your Inner Eaters respond to environmental changes. Stay sensitive to early signals that a part of you is getting triggered.

UPON RETURN:

- **Return to what serves you.** Rather than swinging into restriction, ask, *What would help me feel like myself again?*

- **Prepare for reentry.** Order groceries or plan a nourishing meal to ease the transition back to your normal rhythm.

- **Learn without shame.** If you made choices that didn't feel great, explore what constraints shaped them and how you might navigate similar situations differently.

- **Celebrate adaptation.** Recognize that maintaining some connection to your values while traveling is a victory.

SCENARIO 5. EMOTIONAL EATING, SOLO MEALS, AND ISOLATION

The apartment is quiet. Too quiet. You open the cupboard, then the fridge, then the cupboard again, as if the right food might suddenly materialize.

You're not really hungry, but you're not not-hungry either. You're restless, overstimulated, and ruminating over a difficult conversation. So you grab something—crackers, cookies, that jar of almond butter that's been in cabinet for way too long.

When living alone food easily becomes company. The screen becomes your dining companion. You may eat to mute the volume of your own emotions and drown out the existential loneliness of modern life.

Your Pleasure Eater just wants to feel something nice. Your Survival Eater feels perpetually on edge and food becomes a proxy painkiller. Your Strategic and Social Eaters? Off the grid, silenced, forgotten.

The Eating 2.0 Shift. Get curious about what you *don't want* to feel. Appreciate that your Inner Eaters are trying to comfort you, and food is an easy way to self-soothe. Take responsibility for reengaging with your feelings rather than disconnecting. Explore small ways to feel the hard things before the food numbs it all away.

CONSCIOUS LEADERSHIP STRATEGIES

BEFORE REACHING FOR FOOD:

- **Pause to name the emotion.** Say: *I'm feeling anxious/lonely/ frustrated/excited.*

- **Get curious.** Ask: *What Inner Eater is getting triggered? What is it really asking for? Rest? Celebration? Love?*

- **Explore alternatives.** *Could I tend to this need without food—or with food, but consciously?*
- **Choose intentionally.** If selecting food, do so with awareness. Observe: *I'm choosing this to comfort myself, and I'm okay with that. I will not beat myself up later.*

DURING EMOTIONAL EATING:

- **Create ritual.** Set the table, even for yourself. Use a bowl you like. Bring out fancy silverware or napkins.
- **Slow down.** Sit down, close your eyes, and take one breath before the first bite.
- **Savor taste.** Let your Pleasure Eater receive the gifts of mindful eating.
- **Notice the shift.** How are emotions moving through you? When have you eaten enough?

AFTER THE EXPERIENCE:

- **Avoid self-criticism.** It only perpetuates the cycle, making things worse.
- **Reflect without judgment.** Ask: *Did that meet my need? What else might have helped?*
- **Identify patterns.** Which foods support clean pleasure and which encourage overconsumption?
- **Return to what serves you.** Resume the practices that help you feel integrated—real food, slow eating, home rituals, and strengthening ties.

SCENARIO 6. THE RESTAURANT EXPERIENCE: DINING OUT OR ORDERING IN

You open the menu (or the app) and your brain starts spinning. Sandwiches stacked like architectural feats. Sides large enough to feed four. Cocktails with enough sugar to fuel a marathon.

Your Survival Eater whispers: *"Order big—we don't know when we'll eat like this again."* Your Pleasure Eater is all in: *"This is going to be delicious."* Your Strategic Eater might arrive with a plan: *"I'll have the grilled chicken and vegetables,"* and then become overwhelmed by choice, unsure what tradeoffs are worth making.

This is modern dining in full bloom: an experience designed to maximize excitement and overwhelm you with options. Behind the curtain are behavioral economics nudging you to order more, menu design highlighting the most profitable items, and portions that have nothing to do with what's reasonable.

The old operating system offers two responses.

Option 1. Order everything to "get your money's worth," then feel like you might have overdone it.

Option 2. Over control your order, then feel deprived or overcome with "food envy" while watching others go all-in.

Neither helps you become the eater you want to be.

The Eating 2.0 Shift. Rather than trying to "win" this dining experience, use it as an opportunity to practice leadership in new eating environments. Get curious about what each Inner Eater truly needs in this context. Appreciate that most restaurants are designed to maximize pleasurable consumption, not your health or peace of mind. Take responsibility for leading through the constraints you're facing.

CONSCIOUS LEADERSHIP STRATEGIES

BEFORE YOU GO:

- **Set collaborative intentions.** Choose one nonnegotiable joy (Pleasure Eater's win) and one steady anchor (Strategic Eater's guardrail).

- **Manage your Survival Eater proactively.** Don't arrive ravenous and then panic-order—make choices from centeredness, not desperation.

- **Prepare your Social Eater.** Set realistic expectations about sharing, trying others' food, or navigating group dynamics without abandoning your own needs.

AT THE RESTAURANT:

- **Release the pressure to over optimize.** Aim for choices that feel good enough.

- **Practice both/and decision-making.** Say: *I'll have the pasta I really want* and *pay attention to my satisfaction levels* or *I'll enjoy this indulgent appetizer* and *balance it with a lighter main dish.*

- **Use the meal to practice presence.** Put your fork down between bites, engage in conversation, notice flavors, and develop your capacity to stay present with pleasure.

- **Check in with your Inner Eaters mid meal.** Ask: *Who in me is still hungry? What do we all need right now?*

- **Set kind boundaries.** Acknowledge: *I get to choose what works for me, and I don't need to justify my choices to anyone else.*

AFTER THE MEAL:

- **Appreciate the experience without judgment.** How do you feel physically? Emotionally?

- **Reflect on your leadership.** Did you lead consciously or default to old patterns?

- **Maintain perspective.** One meal doesn't define your relationship with food or derail your health, but every meal is an opportunity to practice conscious choice-making.

- **Extract wisdom for next time.** What lessons could you apply to future dining experiences?

- **Celebrate conscious participation.** Recognize that staying connected to your values while dining out is a victory worth acknowledging.

SCENARIO 7. THE GROCERY STORE GAUNTLET

You walk in for "just a few things." Twenty minutes later, you're halfway through the aisles, slightly dazed, with nothing resembling dinner.

Now you're hungry and your Survival Eater is drooling at the vast abundance of things to eat. Meanwhile, your Pleasure Eater eyes the colorful "NEW" labels, and your Strategic Eater is looking for deals, while clutching to vague health goals.

Welcome to the Food 2.0 shopping experience: candy at the checkout aisle, health halos on ultraprocessed foods, fifty types of milk with no way to determine what is best for your body.

The Eating 2.0 Shift: Get curious about what's captivating your attention. Appreciate that supermarkets are masterclasses in persuasive design created by marketing specialists. Take responsibility for consciously choosing what comes home with you.

CONSCIOUS LEADERSHIP STRATEGIES

BEFORE SHOPPING:

- **Go after meals.** Shopping hungry amplifies impulse purchases.

- **Plan with flexible consistency.** Create a loose list of foods that support your Inner Eaters and actually sound appealing.

- **Give each Inner Eater a voice in the planning process.** Make all parts of you feel included and valued when you step into the store.

IN THE STORE:

- **Shop the perimeter first.** Focus on real foods; read the ingredients, and question bold health claims.

- **Practice the conscious pause.** Before unplanned purchases, ask: *How will this serve my Inner Eaters?*

- **Be selective about Food 2.0 products.** Some may truly add value and convenience to your life; others may just exploit your cravings. Learn to tell the difference.

AFTER SHOPPING:

- **Reflect without judgment.** What did you learn about your Inner Eaters in this environment?

- **Plan improvements.** How could next week's shopping be even more collaborative or harmonious?

- **Celebrate conscious choices.** Recognize that staying connected to your intentions in a grocery store is a significant achievement.

SCENARIO 8. FOOD DESERTS:
WHEN HEALTHY OPTIONS AREN'T AN OPTION

You clock out at 8:00 PM. The gas station is still open, and it is the only place to grab food before tomorrow's 6 AM shift. Fluorescent lights buzz over packaged snacks, energy drinks, and freezer burritos. The "fresh" bananas are brown.

Your Strategic Eater whispers with guilt: "*We should have planned better.*" But the real grocery store is a forty-minute drive away. Your Pleasure Eater doesn't mind. It's been hankering after the hot dog and Cheetos for hours, captivated by Food 2.0 magic.

This is where the dominant food culture becomes most cruel: It promotes a narrow definition of healthy eating while systematically creating food environments that make those choices unavailable. When your nearest place to buy food is only stocked with ultra-processed foods engineered to trigger cravings, the cultural message that you should simply "choose better" becomes not just unhelpful—it's harmful.

The Eating 2.0 Shift. Get curious about the ways the privileged food culture lionizes certain types of eating. Appreciate that your Inner Eaters are working with real constraints, not personal failings. Take responsibility for the choices you can make within the system you're in. Food deserts are systemic flaws. Your Inner Eaters are doing their best within impossible constraints.

CONSCIOUS LEADERSHIP STRATEGIES

BEFORE:

- **Map your grocery store options.** Know what is open, when, how to get there, and if one store has better deals.

- **Stock up when possible.** Load up on shelf-stable real foods that stretch your dollar, like oats, dried beans, rice, canned vegetables, eggs, and so on.

- **Connect with community resources.** Look for food pantries, community gardens, neighbors with different access, and mutual aid.

- **Plan with your constraints.** Ask: *Given my schedule, transportation, and budget, where can I get food for the week?*

DURING:

- **Work the spectrum of processing.** Even with processed options, there are smart choices.

- **Acknowledge your constraints without shame.** Limited options don't make you a limited person.

- **Look for simple combinations.** There are creative ways to pull together a good enough meal at a gas station: perhaps instant oats plus peanut butter, canned beans plus hot sauce, or a bag of frozen peas plus Minute® Rice.

AFTER:

- **Celebrate your resourcefulness.** Note: *I fed myself despite difficult circumstances.*

- **Reflect on systems, not personal failings.** Food deserts are economic and policy failures, not character flaws.

- **Share strategies within your community.** What you've learned about eating well with limited access has value for others facing similar constraints.

- **Channel your frustration toward advocacy.** Your experience gives your credibility to advocate for better access and lobby for healthier options in your community.

SCENARIO 9. CULTURAL FOOD CLASH:
WHEN HERITAGE MEETS WELLNESS CULTURE

You sit across from your mother at Sunday dinner, staring at the dal, rice, and sabzi that anchor every family meal. However, your mind is preoccupied with TikTok wellness influencers, none of whom looked like you or ate food like yours.

Your Strategic Eater has absorbed the message: rice is "bad," carbs are the enemy, real health looks like kale and grass-fed everything. Your Social Eater feels torn between belonging to your family and the influencers you admire. Your Pleasure Eater loves the food and flavors your mother puts into every dish.

You can feel the pull of your old operating system creating false binaries: Either reject your cultural food heritage to fit into social ideals, or abandon health goals to keep the peace at the family table. You're unsure which is worse, falling short of your health goals or disconnecting from your heritage to fit into certain (usually white, western) approaches to food.

The Eating 2.0 Shift. Get curious about the actual nutrition wisdom embedded in your traditional foods. Appreciate that your ancestors developed sophisticated cuisines that sustained them for generations. Take responsibility for defining health on your own terms. Explore how to honor both heritage and your current goals without sacrificing either.

CONSCIOUS LEADERSHIP STRATEGIES

BEFORE:

- **Research your food heritage with pride.** From traditional preparation methods to unique ingredients, there's profound nutrition knowledge in traditional food cultures.

- **Discover the actual nutritional value of your traditional foods.** How much fat is in your grandmother's fried chicken? How much fiber is in your mother's *dal?* How many carbs are in your uncle's *gyoza?*

- **Question wellness culture imperialism.** Ask which wellness messages serve your well-being versus which represent cultural bias or diet culture disguised as health.

- **Connect with others navigating similar cultural-wellness tensions.** Find communities of people honoring their health and heritage without sacrificing either.

DURING:

- **Savor the full experience.** These foods carry flavors, textures, and memories that no mass-produced product can replicate.

- **Engage with food stories.** Ask about family recipes, cooking techniques, or seasonal variations to stimulate conversation about cultural food traditions.

- **Practice flexible consistency.** Your choices can vary widely across different cultural events, family gatherings, and daily life—allow your goals to shift while maintaining a steady shared purpose.

- **Explore thoughtful adaptations.** Add modern foods that you enjoy, adjust portions, or leverage Food 2.0 products to enhance convenience while keeping familiar flavor profiles.

AFTER:

- **Notice how cultural or traditional foods make you feel.** Track your energy, satisfaction, and connection. What worked well for your grandmother's body might not work best for yours.

- **Challenge narrow wellness narratives.** Use your experience and background to educate others about diverse nutrition wisdom and foods they've never tried.

- **Advocate for inclusive wellness.** Support wellness approaches that honor diverse food traditions rather than erase them.

- **Share your story.** Your lived experience can become a model for others navigating similar cultural-wellness tensions.

SCENARIO 10. FEEDING KIDS ON A BUDGET: WHEN EVERYONE NEEDS DIFFERENT THINGS

You stand at the McDonald's counter at 7 PM with your eight-year-old asking for a Happy Meal. You came here because it's between work and soccer practice, and your teenage son only eats chicken nuggets, pizza, and fries anyway. You can feel the familiar pressure building.

Your Strategic Eater calculates cost per meal, trying to make the math work on a tight budget. Your Survival Eater is focused on getting everyone fed quickly before the next activity. You glance back at your daughter, who's already decided she wants the toy that comes with her meal. Meanwhile, your budget wants the value menu, and your mind races with concerns about nutrition.

Your old eating system brings guilt about not cooking "real" food at home, followed by either ordering more expensive, "healthier" options (budget stress) or sticking with what your kids will actually eat (nutrition guilt). You feel like a failing parent either way, standing in a line of other parents making the same impossible calculations.

The Eating 2.0 Shift. Recognize you're facing an enormous challenge: How do you nourish the bodies of your family, teach them life skills, and maintain financial stability while modeling resourcefulness and love? Get curious about what food values you're role-modeling to your kids. Appreciate that feeding a family with limited resources requires advanced-level planning and creativity. Take responsibility for the choices you can make while working to change what you can control.

Your kids need to be fed more than they need perfect nutrition. Love is making sure there's always something to eat. Do the best you can and let that be good enough for today.

CONSCIOUS LEADERSHIP STRATEGIES

BEFORE:

- **Master your family's core menu.** Develop five to seven budget-friendly family meals or restaurants that provide real nutrition that everyone will eat.

- **Research nutrition per dollar.** Find restaurants that offer meal deals for kids. Learn which foods have the most nutritional density and look for those items on menus or sales at the supermarket.

- **Connect with community resources.** Find food banks, community gardens, and other parents sharing strategies for feeding families on tight budgets.

- **Plan with your kids' input.** Explain: "We have X dollars for groceries this week," and ask, "What meals sound good that we could make with that?" This teaches budgeting and gives them a sense of agency.

DURING:

- **Scan options strategically.** Look for combinations that work. For example, protein plus something filling, plus one fun item per kid, rather than trying to optimize everything.

- **Lead by example.** Help your kids understand budgeting, nutrition per dollar, and cooking skills. These are gifts that will serve them for life.

- **If cooking, make it collaborative, not controlling.** Teach the kids how to open cans, stir pots, mix ingredients, or cut veggies. Get them excited about participating in the meal.

AFTER:

- **Acknowledge what went right.** "Everyone ate, we stayed on budget, the kids were happy, and we engaged in conversation."

- **Build on successes rather than dwelling on limitations.** Which meals were hits? Which strategies worked? Which markets have the best deals? Keep those on repeat.

- **Release the guilt.** Remind yourself this is one meal of many, not a referendum on your parenting

Your Personal Field Guide to Eating 2.0

These scenarios provide starting points for a more conscious relationship with food—what I call the Eating 2.0 upgrade. These generic scenarios and canned responses cannot capture the nuance or complexity of your lived reality. Moreover, clinging too tightly to any one of these strategies runs the risk of becoming another impossible ideal to live up to. That defeats the purpose. These suggestions are signposts to what's possible, not standards to judge yourself or others.

EATING 2.0 IN THE REAL WORLD

Your journey through the modern food landscape will be uniquely yours. It's natural to want to "get it right" in a single meal or snack, to judge ourselves on the micro-decisions: *Did I choose the salad or the fries? Did I resist the late-night craving?* But it's crucial not to lose sight of the bigger picture, which is that true health emerges from long-term patterns, not isolated choices.

The real art is holding multiple perspectives: noticing today's meal while remembering that your relationship with food is an evolving journey woven from habits, rituals, and occasional indulgences across weeks, seasons, and a lifetime. As you navigate an ultraprocessed world, remember that every bite counts, but no single bite defines you, and therefore, as you practice Eating 2.0, consider creating your own field notes. Observe:

- What are your top three high-friction eating moments (the times when food decisions feel most challenging or draining)?

- What tensions—such as time pressure, social dynamics, financial constraints, cultural conflicts, or marketing manipulation—make it hard to become the kind of eater you want to be?

- What environments make your eating feel most out of balance?

- Where do you give away your power to Food 2.0 or other people?

Here's the truth: Most Eating 2.0 moments don't feel cinematic. There's no dramatic soundtrack when you choose to eat consciously instead of inhaling food on autopilot. There's no applause when you pause halfway through dinner to check in with yourself. There's no prize for staying connected to your Inner Eaters' wisdom and in charge of their woes. But there is a reward.

The reward is the mental energy that returns when you stop fighting food wars, the emotional steadiness that emerges when you stop oscillating between restriction and rebellion, the physical energy of eating meals that actually satisfy you instead of leaving you searching the pantry an hour later, the profound pleasure of eating like a human being who trusts themself enough to make good food decisions, and the renewed agency to create the life you want rather than what the world of Food 2.0 has plated for you. These are rewards worth fighting for.

Final Thoughts

As our exploration of Eating 2.0 comes to a close, your journey is just beginning. I have a few final ideas I'd like to share about the broader social implications and intangible values of upgrading your eating in an era of existential uncertainty.

EATING AS SACRED PRACTICE AND SOCIAL CONTRIBUTION

The moment you stop fighting your Inner Eaters and start listening to them, something shifts. The constant low-level anxiety about your next meal turns into a reminder to tune in rather than tune out. Your shoulders drop. Your belly softens. You may realize that you've been holding your breath around food for years. Finally, you're returning home to your natural birthright as a participant in the web of life, not an isolated individual consuming nutrients in a late-stage capitalist society.

Although industrial food systems have severed our connection to the source, season, and story of our nourishment, Eating 2.0 weaves those connections back together through conscious daily practice. Every meal becomes an opportunity for embodied presence—giving us a chance to pause our accelerated lives so we may remember that we are not robots to be recharged, but humans in relationship with other living beings, human and nonhuman alike. Relationships are everything, and we must not forget this when we put food in our mouths.

This might look like acknowledging the hands that grew your food or understanding that caring for bodies—yours and others'—is sacred work. It may look like choosing the farmers market tomato over the imported one, or supporting businesses that pay fair wages and reduce food waste, if those options exist. Even if you don't have the financial resources or access to buy sustainably-sourced food, you can model a way of eating that doesn't contribute to body shaming or food moralizing. All of this helps heal Food 2.0's legacy of mindless consumption and social disconnection.

EATING AS FUTURE ANCESTORS FOR YOUNGER GENERATIONS

I have a dream of teaching my son about his Inner Eaters. In fact, I dream of classrooms filled with students learning about their Inner Eaters, so they can better understand themselves, make conscious food choices, and feel empowered to navigate and transform the food systems they've inherited.

Parents who share mindful meals with their children can create bonds extending far beyond the dinner table. Those who embrace their Inner Eaters and model the CARE approach to food have the potential to raise kids who will feel inspired to carry that wisdom forward, and later teach their own children. This is how we collectively upgrade our eating and pass this wisdom down across generations—not through lectures about nutrition, but through the daily demonstration of what it means to eat with the understanding that we are our future descendants' ancestors.

EATING 2.0

THE ONGOING INTEGRATION

Maybe when you started reading this book, you didn't understand how our engineered food systems undermine your natural wisdom about nourishment. It is my hope that you have now discovered that any confusion, cravings, or "noisy" food thoughts you have are not personal failures, but rather your body and mind's adaptations to living in a Food 2.0 environment that profits from your struggle— and mine.

If I have done my job correctly, you now are seeing the modern food landscape with new eyes. I hope you have already started to practice the techniques I've described in this book, especially those of curiosity, appreciation, responsibility, and exploration (CARE). CARE is not a panacea but a way of being with yourself that helps transform food struggles into wisdom.

Ultimately, I'm advocating for wholesome eating—wholesome in the true sense of honoring the whole person you are. This means respecting the full range of your needs: your body's signals, your emotional responses, your social connections, your practical constraints, and yes, your desire for pleasure and convenience. If you can lead your Inner Eaters as a whole, integrated person, then every meal becomes an opportunity to practice presence, compassion, and conscious choice.

Now that you've read this book, I imagine you're different. Not "fixed" or "finished." Now that you are awake to your own motivations, you stand a good chance of becoming the kind of person who can sit at the table with all your contradictions and still choose to feed yourself with integrity. This is what I try to do every day. And even if I miss the mark, I keep trying anyway.

The future needs more people who want to eat with awareness, lead from within, and model a new way forward.

So, go eat.

Eat with care.

Eat with compassion.

Eat like our future depends on it—because it does.

Which leaves only one question: Now that you know who's been eating your lunch . . . what are you going to bring to the table?

EPILOGUE

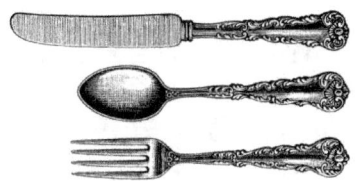

THE DAWN OF EATING 3.0

As I finish writing this book about upgrading our eating, I'm haunted by a terrible irony: We may have spent so much time learning to navigate an era of superabundance that we've for-gotten how to face scarcity.

The Eating 2.0 framework described in these pages, with its emphasis on mindful choices, strategic thinking, and conscious consumption, was designed for a world where the primary challenge was managing overwhelming options—too many calories that are too good to pass up. Food 2.0 requires that we learn to scrutinize hyperpalatable foods, decode marketing messages, and make thoughtful decisions in grocery aisles lined with an inordinate number of products.

But what if that world of obnoxious overabundance is already disappearing?

The children reading this book decades from now may find our concerns quaint—our anxieties about choosing between organic and conventional produce, our debates over meal planning versus intuitive eating, our struggles with food guilt and dietary perfectionism, bemusing them. They might wonder why we spent so much energy learning to navigate choices when choice itself was becoming a luxury they couldn't afford.

Two Futures, One Choice

SCENE ONE: TUESDAY MORNING, 2055

You walk into your kitchen, spit into a machine, and let it scan the stress markers in your saliva. The machine then dispenses your breakfast, a metallic packet. The label promises "Optimized Macro-Nutrient Delivery System," but it tastes like sugared cardboard.

You chew mechanically while your device buzzes with alerts: glucose spike detected, hydration sub-optimal, mood-enhancement supplement recommended for $47.99.

At the grocery store, dim lights buzz over half-empty shelves. A few staples remain—powdered lentil flour, algae paste, fortified soy milk—but they're rationed. A wall-mounted screen scans your biometric ID and flashes: "Protein quota met for the week."

No one lingers. People shuffle through like it's a clinic, not a market. You receive assigned sustenance, eyes hollow. Real food is rare. Real joy, rarer. Outside, a billboard reads: "Eat responsibly. The planet depends on you."

SCENE TWO: TUESDAY MORNING, 2055

You step into the edible heart of your neighborhood, not a store, but a living ecosystem. Raised beds brim with purple bok choy and fragrant herbs. Kids weave between garden rows; their fingers stained with blackberry juice.

Inside the food co-op, sunlight pours through solar glass. An AI dashboard displays this week's nutrient yields and soil health scores. Your wristband suggests: "You're low on magnesium. Consider the sweet potato and kale stew tonight." You receive a basket of ingredients harvested that morning—zero waste, zero packaging.

Along the wall, a culinary apprentice learns sourdough techniques from a seventy-three-year-old baker who still measures by feel. In the community classroom, third graders compare macronutrients in beans and bugs. Then they taste test both with curiosity, not disgust.

Here, eating isn't just about survival; it's how people learn, bond, and grow. Food is woven into the fabric of education, civic life, and ecological stewardship.

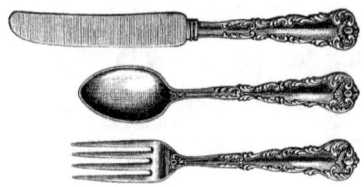

IN ONE FUTURE, eating is a problem to be solved. In the other, eating is connection to be cultivated.

The path we choose—individually and collectively—will determine which story we live. And that choice begins right now.

Feast or Famine?
The Future of Eating

Food 1.0 was our ancestral dance with seasonal abundance and scarcity that lasted for millennia. The first great transition—Food 1.5—emerged with the dawn of agriculture. Humans began to sow, reap, herd, and store. Gradually, food became less a matter of daily chance and more a product of planning and cultivation. Food 2.0, which accelerated with industrialization in the twentieth century, introduced caloric surplus, engineered hyper-palatability, and constant availability. Although rich, industrialized nations are still living in the conspicuous consumption of a Food 2.0 era, its time may be coming to an end. Sooner or later, what we recognize as food and take for granted as "normal" eating will be a relic of the past. Food 2.0 will fade away, and Food 3.0 will emerge, promising something entirely different: a convergence of crisis and innovation that will fundamentally reshape not just what we eat, but how we think about eating itself.

Multiple seismic shifts are colliding to create this next stage. Climate change is redrawing the agricultural map, turning breadbaskets into deserts while opening new growing regions in previously frozen territories. Global supply chains are feeling increasingly fragile, subject to widespread crop failures and diseases, as well as shipping logjams and even piracy. Meanwhile, consumers demand transparency, sustainability, and health outcomes that current food corporations struggle to deliver (or would prefer not to deliver).

Technology is accelerating these changes at an unprecedented pace. Lab-grown meat is transitioning from science fiction to grocery store reality. Present-day 3D food printers will move from research labs into home kitchens. Precision fermentation will create dairy proteins without cows, and eggs without chickens. The very definition of *food* will expand to include creations incomprehensible to previous generations.

Perhaps most dramatically, pharmaceutical interventions like GLP-1 agonists will continue to decouple hunger from habit, appetite from addiction. For the first time in human history, we're developing tools that directly modulate our fundamental drive to eat—a philosophical earthquake forcing us to reconsider the role of desire, restraint, and choice in our relationship with food.

The Emergence of Food 3.0

If Food 2.0 was ultraprocessed, Food 3.0 will be precision-engineered, characterized by radical personalization and severe environmental constraints. Mass production will give way to mass customization at the cellular level. These foods will be designed for precise physiological outcomes, such as increasing muscle protein synthesis, supporting specific beneficial bacteria, and enhancing cognition and immunity.

Food 3.0 will likely be produced in labs, vertical farms, or cellular agriculture facilities. Global supply chains will contract and have to be relocated by the people who operate them due to climate change, water scarcity, and shifting political borders. Expect more mycelium protein, microalgae, and insect-based ingredients to become quietly integrated into our everyday staples.

This technological marvel will bring new challenges to future eaters. They will face entirely new decisions, like:

- *Should I eat algae-based protein optimized for my workout or fermented cricket flour designed to support my gut microbiome?*

- *How do I balance the environmental impact of my mycelium burger against its glucose response?*

- *Does this protein source support my genetic markers for longevity while meeting my carbon budget?*

- *Will choosing the inflammation-reducing option conflict with my weekly microplastic limits?*

- *Do I take hunger-mitigating drugs or satiety shakes and skip eating altogether?*

Today's Strategic Eater already feels overwhelmed trying to balance organic versus local, low-carb versus Mediterranean, and determining whether a particular "superfood" label is marketing or science. By 2055, this complexity will explode exponentially. Every food choice will carry cascading implications, and the cognitive burden of evaluating nutritional content, environmental impact, and ethical implications with every food choice will be enormous.

The Social Transformation of Eating

The social fabric of eating is already fraying and reweaving itself. The traditional three-meal structure, already weakened by the rise of snacking culture, may fragment entirely as personalized nutrition demands precise meal timing. You won't eat because it's lunch or because you feel hungry. You will eat—or consume concocted nutrients—because it's the biologically optimal time to feed your cells and microbiome.

Dining out will bifurcate into two radically different experiences.

"Heritage houses" will emerge as ultra-high-end culinary museums where traditional cooking becomes cultural preservation. These establishments will employ food historians alongside chefs, serving dishes requiring human hands and time-intensive techniques. A meal might cost the same as a month's groceries but offer something increasingly rare: sensory memory of how humans ate for millennia.

"Nutrition hubs" will dominate everyday dining—sleek spaces resembling pharmacies more than restaurants. You'll scan your biometric ID and receive precisely calibrated meals designed for your current metabolic state. The food might be 3D-printed, optimized for absorption and glycemic response, technically food

—perfectly balanced, sustainably produced, allergen-free—but tasting like fuel.

Between these extremes, casual restaurants offering imperfect food at reasonable prices may become economically unsustainable. The middle-class ritual of "going out to dinner" could become as obsolete as gathering around the radio.

This stark division in social eating may also catalyze a counter-movement away from dystopian extremes or elite eating establishments. Community kitchens and food cooperatives might emerge as a third way forward. There could be spaces where people gather to cook and eat together using both traditional techniques and new technologies, reclaiming the social aspects of cooking that both the Heritage Houses and Nutrition Hubs fail to provide. These grassroots alternatives could become the most important dining innovation of all, proving that the future of eating out doesn't have to choose between nostalgia and optimization, but can integrate both in the service of human connection.

The Disappearance of Grocery Shopping

Grocery shopping may soon feel like a relic. Imagine stepping into a market in 2055: dim lights conserving energy, half-empty shelves from supply disruptions like severe bird flu, drought, and massive flooding. Where there were once forty-seven kinds of granola on display, now there are three: one optimized for blood sugar, one for climate impact, and one for national policy compliance.

In affluent zones, grocery shopping may become hyper-digitized. Wealthy consumers will print meals at home, receive AI-optimized ingredient pods, and consult embedded AI kitchen dietitians. The gap between those with personalized nutrition and those with mass-produced alternatives may define future inequality.

Subscription services will sync biometric data and planetary impact scores to generate meal plans. Ingredients might even arrive in tubes via drone. Packaging could become edible, or, at the very least, compostable in your own home. Food waste could become obsolete as production matches consumption with algorithmic precision. Think of it as the natural evolution of what we're already seeing today—your smartwatch tracking your steps and sleep, meal kit services like HelloFresh delivering pre-portioned ingredients, and apps like MyFitnessPal logging your nutrition. The difference is that by 2055, these separate systems will merge into one seamless experience where your morning health metrics automatically adjust your evening grocery delivery, eliminating both the guesswork of "What's for dinner?" and the guilt of throwing away wilted lettuce you forgot about in your fridge.

Older generations will lament over what has been lost. Gone is the joyful chaos of shopping carts bumping in Trader Joe's. Gone is the sensory pleasure of sniffing peaches or inspecting your eggs. Gone is the decision of whether to pack up leftovers or clean your plate. The simple pleasure of choosing from shelves of imperfect, inefficient, but deeply satisfying foods will be nostalgia.

If the purchasing of food becomes increasingly centralized and regulated, a black market may flourish, selling blacklisted ingredients, heritage seeds, or contraband items. Imagine cheeses banned due to their carbon footprints or chocolate restricted for its water usage. Underground dinner parties might serve "illegal" beef or unregulated heirloom tomatoes that don't meet government standards.

The questions then become, *What do I do with this delicious cheese I got on the black market if my biometric device is tracking* everything I consume? How do I skirt the algorithmically enforced fat limits? How do I bypass the public-health mandated caloric cap?

Food 3.0 may be far more policed and more political than we're used to today—infinitely customizable and frictionless, but oddly *soulless*.

The Emergence of Eating 3.0

If Eating 2.0 emerged as a conscious act of reclaiming peace, purpose, and power in abundant food landscapes, then Eating 3.0 will be defined by adaptation to technological mediation, climate instability, and regulated rationing. Future eaters will likely contend with strict policies, supply limitations, and health optimization beyond anything we've seen.

Just as people have fallen into autopilot eating or dieting, future eaters will likely have to choose between two paths: completely outsourcing their eating to algorithms and government-subsidized Food 3.0 or getting swept up in overwhelming personalized optimization that promises health while losing joy, spontaneity, and social bonding.

Traditional wisdom like "Eat when hungry, stop when full" loses meaning when hunger can be chemically modulated and satiation precisely controlled. "Eat real food" becomes meaningless if algae burgers are indistinguishable from beef burgers. "Cook from scratch" will sound quaint when your kitchen AI can synthesize any flavor profile from base nutrients in minutes, making a three-hour marinara sauce seem as obsolete as churning butter by hand.

As eating becomes medicalized and technologized, we may forget how to *feel* our way through our food choices. Think about how GPS has already made us lose our sense of direction, or how autocorrect weakens our spelling instincts. When biofeedback-regulated, pre-portioned solutions become faster and cheaper, we'll decouple eating from intuition. The pleasure of eating your grandmother's soup on a rainy day or sharing a spontaneous late-night pizza with friends is a deeply human experience that may fade. Eating will become a purely functional activity if food is optimized for our bodies like fuel for a machine. But in losing the messiness, the mistakes, the discovery of eating experiences, we would risk losing something essential about what makes us human: the rich tapestry of memory, culture, and relationship that eating weaves through our lives.

When the Ritual Disappears: The Collapse of Food Identity

Who are you when your way of eating no longer exists?

Let's say that you were raised in Texas in the 2020s with mesquite smoke and brisket pride. In the good old days, the pitmaster was like a priest, presiding over a meat communion. But in 2055, cattle now costs the same as caviar by weight. Ranchland has turned to dust. A pound of real beef is more sought after than designer watches or handbags. Most meat is vat-grown, engineered by neural networks trained on old taste archives. What happens to you, the Texan eater, when there's no cow, no fire, no grill?

In Japan, by 2055 the collapse is quieter but no less profound. The sushi chef—once a symbol of artistic precision and generational mastery—now serves fermented kelp cubes and jellyfish extract. Bluefin tuna are extinct. The bigeye are too loaded with mercury and plastic to consume. Ocean fisheries have collapsed due to acidification. You still have your grandfather's hand-carved chopsticks, but there's nothing delicate left to pick up.

What will happen to a culture that once defined beauty through the art of eating when the art is obsolete? Where would the chopsticks go in a test-tube world of Food 3.0? Perhaps you will be able to find those wooden relics in the Grocery Store Museum next to the sensory immersion pods that simulate the thick aromas of a Texas smokehouse.

The Inner Eaters of the Future

How will our internal family system of Eaters adapt to these external forces? Will new tools strengthen our Inner Eaters capacity to respond or degrade them entirely? While I cannot predict what will happen, I can speculate on the Inner Eaters of the future. I imagine that:

The Survival Eater will bifurcate. On one hand, it will be coddled by data-driven nutrient delivery that ensures hunger never arises. The felt sense of needing to eat may become technologically or medically eradicated. On the other hand, the Survival Eater will, in fact, be eating for survival. It may become hypervigilant because of food shortages and severe restrictions. When tomorrow's meal is not guaranteed, it will clamor after any food it can find.

The Pleasure Eater will fracture. On one hand, ever-more engineered eating experiences will threaten to hijack every pleasure chemical in our bodies. We will need to establish clear boundaries for it, lest we become addicted to the "high". On the other hand, the Pleasure Eater will end up feeling completely neglected by bland vitamin slurries and drab nutrient shakes that deliver calories without mouth appeal—fuel devoid of joy.

The Social Eater will rebuild new rituals. Family dinner may be replaced by gathering around the 3D printer, watching it stitch and layer perfectly portioned proteins. Yet when each person at the table has different nutritional needs and chemically modulated appetites, it will become harder to share food. Your teenager's metabolism-optimized pasta won't match your spouse's heart-health formula, and Grandma's memory-enhancement meal will bear no resemblance to your toddler's brain-development blend. The communal act of passing dishes, stealing bites from each other's plates, or cooking one big pot that everyone enjoys will fragment into individual, personalized experiences—physically together but nutritionally isolated. More people will eat with AI personalities or robot humanoids that don't require any food at all.

The Strategic Eater will become challenged. It will struggle to navigate complex landscapes of nutrient claims, planetary pleas, and disease-proof necessities. It will likely morph into a Techno-Strategic Eater, relying on algorithms and apps to guide (and override) food choices. Massive education and digital literacy will be necessary to interpret the onslaught of health advice and personalized data. Many people will feel helpless without their technological intermediaries (and perhaps nostalgic for the days when choosing an apple was just about whether it looked ripe.)

The Rise of the Ecological Eater

Climate realities may birth an entirely new Inner Eater demanding a louder voice: the Ecological Eater. People who adhere to the urges of the Ecological Eater will track food miles like macros, count water usage alongside calories, and evaluate meals by their impact on soil biodiversity and carbon sequestering. Being driven by this eater means taking food production into your own hands with the urgency that previous generations never felt.

Your kitchen may become your micro-farm, windows lined with sprouting trays, countertops crowded with fermentation vessels, and every available surface nurturing something edible. Backyards will be rewilded into food forests where fruit trees, mushroom logs, and pollinator gardens create ecosystems rather than lawns. The Ecological Eater might drive you to join community land shares, participate in seed swaps, or learn skills your great-grandparents took for granted—preserving, fermenting, and storing food seasonally.

When heeding this voice, you will shift from asking *What do I want to eat?* to *What does the world need me to eat?* as increasingly complex implications for the environment, global equity, animal welfare, and our own health are in the balance.

People who default to this lens will eat as an act of planetary citizenship. They will want to know if this food or that food is good for the world they are leaving their children. *Did those almonds drain our aquifers? Does this tomato support regenerative farming practices? How many animals thrived or suffered to bring this meal to my plate?* Every bite will carry a moral weight. A burger won't be judged by taste or protein alone, but by the pasture it came from, the methane it produced, and the hands that raised it.

The Ecological Eater will scan QR codes revealing the carbon journey of every ingredient, from seed to disposal. But it won't stop at there. For many, ecological eating will become an identity as significant as their religion or political affiliation. Some may embrace modern animism, extending ethical consideration to plants, fungi, and microbes. Others may reclaim some premodern rituals and revere eating as magical energetic transmutation— sacred moments where one life becomes another.

From this worldview, new food-based spiritual movements will bloom. Ancient traditions may resurface, reviving Indigenous reciprocity practices, seasonal fasting cycles, or offerings to land spirits that acknowledge our interdependence with soil and water. Entirely novel practices will emerge alongside these revivals:

311

climate monasteries growing zero-carbon diets; neomonastic urban communes where members pledge to consume only foods that restore more than they deplete. New religious movements may bless certain foods while prohibiting others based on their environmental and ethical footprints. The eco-agro religions of the future will be a wild west of competing carbon commandments and nitrogen-cycle prophets. The most orthodox sects will require members to memorize the carbon footprint of every ingredient, like scripture. At the same time, progressive branches will allow carbon offsets as a form of dietary indulgence—proving that even when we try to save the planet through spiritual eating, we'll still find ways to make it complicated, contradictory, and surprisingly capitalist.

The Reclamation of Meaning

The future challenges us: What do we preserve when the world says our ways of eating must change?

When cheap beef disappears, can the grill master find new life in mesquite-roasted eggplants or algae burgers? When fish vanish, can sushi reverence redirect toward seaweed biodiversity? When Thanksgiving arrives, will it return to home-cooked abundance or disappear in food scarcity scrambles?

These questions pull at my heartstrings and knot my stomach. But here's the flicker of hope, the stubborn ember I can't extinguish: Maybe this work of upgrading our eating to Eating 2.0—the internal integration, external intentionality, conscious leadership over our Inner Eaters—isn't destined to become obsolete. Maybe it's exactly what the future demands, humans capable of matching novel eating challenges with sophistication and integrity. Maybe it's the warmup, the necessary upgrade before the even bigger overhaul.

EATING 2.0

The next phase of eating will be shaped by technology and necessity, but it must also be shaped by *leadership and imagination*. Can we bravely lead our Inner Eaters into the future of eating? Can we allow them to transform us into the eaters *we need to become*? Can we imagine new foods and new ways of eating that still feel good, true, and beautiful in a world that's hard to recognize?

The dinner table of 2055 may look nothing like ours today, but no matter what happens—whether food becomes pill, paste, or printed macros—the inner terrain remains. Who we are as eaters will always be as essential to our relationship with food as what we're eating. Our basic human need for physical, emotional, and social nourishment stays constant despite what Food 3.0 has in store.

Our challenge is to ensure that in all our technological sophistication, we don't forget to feed the whole human being. If we've done this work—learned to listen inward with care and creatively inhabit constraints and contradictions of our food environment—we'll carry forward something no system collapse can erase: the choice to feed each other with intention, to eat with reverence, to remember that every bite connects us to the web of life that sustains us all.

Although the future may not let us eat as we once did, somewhere in the space between what we've lost and what we're becoming lies the human power to care for each other through sharing food. Cooking for others can transform even mundane meals into acts of love, and although that might not be enough to ward off famine or disaster, it's the thread that I am holding onto, in the hopes that it will weave us back together when everything else falls apart.

ACKNOWLEDGMENTS

I would like to take this opportunity to thank the many people and influences that helped to shape this book. While the ideas in the book may be expressed through words of my choosing, they are not "mine" in any real sense. They are built upon notions, frameworks, research, and wisdom from countless others, as much as they are based on my personal experiences of eating in a Food 2.0 world. I will attempt to give credit where it is due, but no matter how hard I try, this list will be woefully incomplete.

MOTHER EARTH

Beyond the brilliant minds that came before me is Nature herself. My deepest attribution goes to the land: Mother Earth, Pachamama, Gaia, this incredible blue biosphere we call home. We are an extension of you. With deep reverence, I reap the ideas contained within these pages from your soil, and I eat your gifts with utmost gratitude.

FAMILY

To my dad, who has been with me every step of this journey. From our earliest discussions of a book while scribbling ideas on cocktail napkins to your red-pen edits of later drafts, you've been a thought partner, anchor, and champion. I can't thank you enough for your guidance.

To my mom, my number one fan, for encouraging me to stay the course and bring this book to fruition.

ACKNOWLEDGMENTS

To Asher, I hope this book helps you better understand who I was before I became your father and brings you and your generation new ideas, tools, and strategies for eating well.

To Claire, for putting up with my early mornings and late nights of writing. Multiple times I felt frustrated and discouraged, and the many pep talks you gave me—encouraging me to keep writing and not give up—carried me through. I love you.

FRIENDS AND CLIENTS

To Pete Kadushin for ping-ponging ideas, blasting them into outer space, and reeling them back to reality. Your thought partnership has been invaluable.

To Mike Davidson for being an early advocate of the Inner Eaters and allowing me to test drive frameworks through your lived experience.

To Soltan Bryce for ongoing friendship and support, encouraging me to let the writing unfold and not force the book to bend to my timeline. It has marinated. I have grown. Here's the better, juicer version that came about because of you.

To Drew Nelson for being a thought partner, soul brother, and level five master improviser. Your astute mind and humor have kept me noodling on what matters most and have inspired me to stay true to my values and ethics.

To many other friends who cheered for me during this journey, showed interest in the topic, and helped me clarify what I was communicating. Abe, Mari, Chantal, Dave, and others, you've made this book better, and I can't thank you enough.

To all my clients: Your vulnerability and openness allowed me to see "under the hood" of your eating and discover the patterns and parts that have now become the Inner Eaters. I want to thank you for working with me and tolerating me when I said, "I should really put this in a book someday." Well, here it is!

EDITORIAL AND BUSINESS PARTNERSHIP

To Stephanie Gunning, my amazing editor, who walked with me on this journey from concept to completion through hesitation, self-doubt, uncertainty, excitement, and every possible space in between. Thank you for continuing to work with me line by line to bring this book to life.

To Kate Sedrowski, who has supported me since the earliest days swinging through BKB to recent years of online coaching. Your partnerships and assistance with all things "web" have made it possible to grow and evolve my coaching practice. Without you, I'd be fumbling through MailChimp, chasing my own tail. Thank you for bringing your design skills and warm heart to everything we've worked on together—let's ascend to new heights and grab a meal at the top!

TEACHERS AND MENTORS

The work of many teachers, coaches, and guides, living and dead, contributed to my thinking as I was writing this book. In truth, they are too numerous to name. I've gained tremendous wisdom from the books, videos, and podcasts of some I've never even met. In no particular order, I want to acknowledge key influences that have shaped my thinking and relationship with food.

Mark David, thank you for the unrivaled Dynamic Eating Psychology training. You planted the seeds of these concepts years ago by asking me "who" was doing the eating. Your guidance and wisdom have been invaluable.

ACKNOWLEDGMENTS

Metta McGarvey, you're an incredible teacher, friend and copilot, and I owe so many of these ideas to you and our work together. Thank you for helping me continue to find my wholeness.

A special thanks to Jamie Wheal for teaching me how to write books that people actually want to read.

Ken Wilber and the entire Integral Life community, your ideas continue to percolate in my consciousness, stir in my soul, and help me try to wrap my mind around the dizzying complexity of life as we know it (while also letting go of the idea that I'll ever really understand the great mystery).

Augusto Pinaud, thanks for being so excited about this book, even when the ideas were admittedly half baked. Your support and encouragement were essential in getting this to completion.

Keith Martin-Smith, Nitzan Hermon, and Carlos Manuel Egaña, your sage wisdom, caring feedback, and precise prompting helped me grow and expand my thinking. I appreciate the ways you challenged and supported me.

My gratitude also extends to:

Richard C. Schwartz for clarifying how our mind is made up of distinct sub-personalities or "parts" that interact with each other. Thank you for pioneering integrated systems thinking and bringing this work to the mainstream.

David Peter Stroh and Donella Meadows for the exemplary work on complexity.

Fariha Roisin and Chrissy King, for opening my eyes to the racialized and classist injustices of the wellness world.

Bee Willson, for your wonderful books and food advocacy.

Valarie Kaur for being a heartfelt hero, leading with revolutionary love.

Caroline Myss and Terry Patten for wisdom from beyond that stimulated my spiritual sensibilities.

For teaching me how to reclaim my pleasure, adrienne maree brown.

Michael Pollan and Mark Bittman for your ongoing thought leadership and advocacy for a more just food system.

David L. Katz, M.D., for continuing to be a voice of sanity and clarity in a wellness world ripe with misinformation.

Others who have profoundly influenced this work include Paul Chek, Peter Attia, Daniel Siegel, Mary O'Malley, Steven Kotler, Robert Kegan, James Carse, William Li, Clare W. Graves, Abraham Maslow, Pooja Lakshmin, Christy Harrison, Andrew Weil, Chris van Tulleken, Paco Underhill, Chip Heath, Sophie Egan, Mark Hyman, David Kessler, Michelle Segar, Sumner Brooks, Amee Severson, Evelyn Tribole, and Elyse Resch, and many more whose ideas have inspired and shaped me across the years.

THE INVISIBLE HANDS

I want to thank every person whose invisible hand ever has played a role in feeding me: from watering seeds to picking vegetables, packaging them in facilities, driving them in freight trucks, unloading them in supermarkets, and stocking shelves. The labor and effort of those helping me check out at the market is not forgotten. For making meals, and doing the dishes, I am grateful to the outstanding chefs, cooks, and other kitchen staff from the many restaurants where I have dined. Thank you, one and all, for helping keep me fed, alive, and nourished.

NOTES

Preface

1. N. Auger, B.J. Potter, U.V. Ukah, et al. (2021). "Anorexia Nervosa and the Long-term Risk of Mortality in Women," *World Psychiatry*, vol. 20, no.3 (September 9, 2021): pp. 448–9.

Introduction

1. "The Flavorists: Tweaking Tastes and Creating Cravings," YouTube video, posted by CBS News, September 2, 2012.
2. *The Cheesecake Factory Nutritional Guide 2.25* (retrieved February 17, 2025, from TheCheesecakeFactory.com).
3. Norman P. Li, Mark van Vugt, and Stephen M. Colarelli. "The Evolutionary Mismatch Hypothesis: Implications for Psychological Science," *Current Directions in Psychological Science*, vol. 27, no.1 (2018): pp. 38–44. Also *see*, William W. Li. *Eat to Beat Disease: The New Science of How Your Body Can Heal Itself* (New York: Grand Central Publishing, 2019).

PART ONE

Chapter 1: How Food2.0 Hijacks What You Eat

Epigraph. Michael Moss. *Salt Sugar Fat: How the Food Giants Hooked Us* (New York: Random House Publishing Group, 2013): p. 147.
1. Joe Bubar. "Do Junk Food Ads Make You Hungry?" *New York Times Upfront*, Scholastic.com (January 4, 2021).

2. Robert H. Lustig. "Ultraprocessed Food: Addictive, Toxic, and Ready for Regulation," *Nutrients*, vol. 12, no. 11 (November 5, 2020): article 3401.

3. Tera L. Fazzino, Daiil Jun, Lynn Cholett-Hinton, et al. "US Tobacco Companies Selectively Disseminated Hyperpalatable Foods into the US Food System: Empirical Evidence and Current Implications." *Addiction*, vol. 119, no. 1 (January 2024): pp. 62–71.

4. Wei Wu, Jiawei Zhou, Rongrong Xuan, et al. (2022). Dietary κ-Carrageenan Facilitates Gut Microbiota-mediated Intestinal Inflammation," *Carbohydrate Polymers*, vol. 277 (February 1, 2022): e118830. Also *see*, Andrea Petersen. "Emulsifiers Make Food More Appealing. Do They Also Make You Sick?" *Wall Street Journal* (March 3, 2025).

5. John O. Warner. "Artificial Food Additives: Hazardous to Long-term Health?" *Archives of Disease in Childhood*, vol. 109, no. 11 (October 18, 2024): pp. 882–5.

6. Veronique Bouvard, Dana Loomis, Kathryn Z. Guyton, et al. (IARC Working Group). "Carcinogenicity of Consumption of Red and Processed Meat." *Lancet Oncology*, vol. 16, no. 16 (December 2015): pp. 1599–1600.

7. Mathilde Touvier, Maria Loura da Costa Louzada, Dariush Mozaffarian, et al. "Ultraprocessed Foods and Cardiometabolic Health: Public Health Policies to Reduce Consumption Cannot Wait," *BMJ*, vol. 383 (October 9, 2023): e075294.

8. "Ultraprocessed Foods: My Verdict," LinkedIn.com, posted by David L. Katz, MD, MPH, January 17, 2025.

9. Susan E. Swithers. "Artificial Sweeteners Produce the Counterintuitive Effect of Inducing Metabolic Derangements," *Trends in Endocrinology and Metabolism*, vol. 24, no. 9 (September 2013): pp. 431–41.

10. Michael Moss. *Salt Sugar Fat: How the Food Giants Hooked Us* (New York: Random House Publishing Group, 2013).

11. David J. Linden. *The Compass of Pleasure: How Our Brains Make Fatty Foods, Orgasm, Exercise, Marijuana, Generosity, Vodka, Learning, and Gambling Feel So Good* (New York: Penguin Books, 2011): pp. 24-25.

12. Ruben Nogueiras, Amparo Romero-Picó, Maria J. Vazquez, et al. "The Opioid System and Food Intake: Homeostatic and Hedonic Mechanisms." *Obesity Facts*, vol. 5, no. 2 (April 19, 2012): pp. 196–207.

13. Andrew Huberman. "Protocols for Excellent Parenting and Improving Relationships of All Kinds | Dr. Becky Kennedy," YouTube video, posted by Andrew Huberman, February 26, 2024.

14. Sarah Zhang. "Americans Don't Really Like to Chew," TheAtlantic.com (July 7, 2023).

15. Tera L. Fazzino, Amber B. Courville, Juen Guo, et al. "Ad Libitum Meal Energy Intake Is Positively Influenced by Energy Density, Eating Rate and Hyper-palatable Food Across Four Dietary Patterns," *Nature Food*, vol. 4, no. 2 (January 30, 2023): pp. 144–7.

16. Clinical Center News. "First Randomized, Controlled Study Finds Ultra-processed Diet Leads to Weight Gain," NIH.gov (July 1, 2019).

17. Kevin D. Hall, Alexis Ayuketah, Robert Brychta, et al. "Ultra-Processed Diets Cause Excess Calorie Intake and Weight Gain: An Inpatient Randomized Controlled Trial of Ad Libitum Food Intake," *Cell Metabolism*, vol. 30, no. 1 (July 2, 2019): pp. 67–77, E3.

18. Ibid.

19. Stephen A. Witherly. *Why Humans Like Junk Food: The Inside Story on Why You Like Your Favorite Foods, the Cuisine Secrets of Top Chefs, and How to Improve Your Own Cooking Without a Recipe!* (Lincoln, NE.: iUniverse, 2007): p. 12.

20. Daisuke Hayashi, Caitlyn Edwards, Jennifer A. Emond, et al. "What Is Food Noise? A Conceptual Model of Food Cue Reactivity," *Nutrients*, vol. 15, no. 22 (November 17, 2023): e4809.

21. Barbara J. Rolls, Erin L. Morris, and Liane S. Roe. "Portion Size of Food Affects Energy Intake in Normal-weight and Overweight Men and Women," *American Journal of Clinical Nutrition*, vol. 76, no. 6 (December 2022): pp. 1207–13.

22. Lisa R. Young and Marion Nestle. "The Contribution of Expanding Portion Sizes to the US Obesity Epidemic," *American Journal of Public Health*, vol. 92, no. 2 (February 2002): pp. 246–9.

23. Ashleigh Haynes, Charlotte A. Hardman, Alexis D.J. Makin, et al. "Visual Perceptions of Portion Size Normality and Intended Food Consumption: A Norm Range Model," *Food Quality and Preference*, vol. 72 (March 2019): pp. 77–85.

24. Florence Sheen, Charlotte A. Hardman, and Eric Robinson. "Plate-clearing Tendencies and Portion Size Are Independently Associated with Main Meal Food Intake in Women: A Laboratory Study," *Appetite*, vol. 127 (August 2018): pp. 223–9.

25. The idea that as portions grow, so does consumption seems to be true up to a point. Once portions violate preconceptions of normality people will adjust their consumption downward to compensate. However, there a appears to be a large range of what one deems normal. This allows significant wiggle room for eating to expand as portions grow.

26. Paul Rozin, Kimberly Kabnick, Erin Pete, et al. "The Ecology of Eating: Smaller Portion Sizes in France Than in the United States Help Explain the French Paradox," *Psychological Science*, vol. 14, no. 5 (September 2003): pp. 450–4.

27. American Academy of Pediatrics Committee on Nutrition. "Changes to the Nutrition Facts Label: What Parents Need to Know," HealthyChildren.org (last updated April 23, 2020).

28. Barry Schwartz. *The Paradox of Choice: Why More Is Less, Revised Edition* (New York: HarperCollins Publishers, 2009).

29. Richard J. Johnson, Mark S. Segal, Yuri Sautin, et al. "Potential Role of Sugar (Fructose) in the Epidemic of Hypertension, Obesity and the Metabolic Syndrome, Diabetes, Kidney Disease, and Cardiovascular Disease," *American Journal of Clinical Nutrition*, vol. 86, no. 4 (October 2007): pp. 899–906.

30. It's important to note that the term *calorie availability* refers to the average amount of food energy available per person per day, which includes both consumption and food waste. Therefore, actual caloric intake may be lower than availability figures suggest. *See*, Joyce H. Lee, Miranda Duster, Timothy Roberts, et al. "United States Dietary Trends Since 1800: Lack of Association Between Saturated Fatty Acid Consumption and Non-communicable Diseases," *Frontiers in Nutrition*, vol. 8 (January 12, 2022): e748847.

31. GBD 2021 US Obesity Forecasting Collaborators. "National-level and State-level Prevalence of Overweight and Obesity Among Children, Adolescents, and Adults in the USA, 1990–2021, and Forecasts up to 2050," *Lancet*, vol. 404, no. 10469: pp. 2278–98.

32. Ryan Andrews. "All about Kitchen Makeovers," PrecisionNutrition.com (accessed June 17, 2025).

NOTES

Chapter 2: When Dinner Broke

Epigraph. Ellen Cushing. "How Snacks Took over American Life," TheAtlantic.com (September 6, 2024).

1. Karen Hamrick and Ket McClelland. "Americans' Eating Patterns and Time Spent on Food: The 2014 Eating & Health Module Data," Economic Research Service, U.S. Department of Agriculture (July 2016): p.13.

2. U.S. Department of Health and Human Services and U.S. Department of Agriculture. (2020). "Part D. Chapter 13: Frequency of Eating," *Scientific Report of the 2020 Dietary Guidelines Advisory Committee* (July 2020).

3. Cushing.

4. U.S. Department of Agriculture. "Food Expenditure Series—Interactive Charts," Economic Research Service, U.S. Department of Agriculture (updated June 3, 2025). Food Expenditure Series - Interactive Charts: Food Expenditures

5. I performed calculations based on information found on the following website. Economic Research Service, U.S. Department of Agriculture. "National Food Expenditure Series–Interactive Charts: Food Expenditures," ERS.USDA.gov (updated June 3, 2025).

6. Jerry Gillam. "California Elections: Proposition 163: Lawmakers Keeping Quiet on Repeal of Snack Tax,' *Los Angeles Times* (October 29, 1992).

7. Jan-Emmanuel De Neve, Andrew Dugan, Micah Kaats, et al. "Sharing Meals with Others: How Sharing Meals Supports Happiness and Social Connections," *World Happiness Report 2025* (accessed June 23, 2025).

8. Eric Robinson, Paul Aveyard, Amanda Daley, et al. "Eating Attentively: A Systematic Review and Meta-analysis of the Effect of Food Intake Memory and Awareness on Eating,"

American Journal of Clinical Nutrition, vol. 97, no. 4 (April 2013): pp. 728–42.

9. Jennifer L. Harris, Frances Fleming-Milici, Sally Mancini, et al. "Rudd Report: Targeted Food and Beverage Advertising to Black and Hispanic Consumers: 2022 Update," Rudd Center for Food Policy and Health, University of Connecticut (November 2022).

10. Marc David. "Emotional Eating and Pleasure: What's the Connection?" Institute for the Psychology of Eating (August 28, 2023).

11. Y.H.C. Yau, and M.N. Potenza. "Stress and Eating Behaviors," *Minerva Endocrinologica*, vol. 38, no. 3 (September 2013): pp. 255–67.

12. Kristen L. Knutson and Eve Van Cauter. "Associations Between Sleep Loss and Increased Risk of Obesity and Diabetes," *Annals of the New York Academy of Sciences*, vol. 1129, no. 1 (June 28, 2018): pp. 287–304.

13. Isabel E. Young, Amudha Poobalan, Katherine Steinbeck, et al. "Distribution of Energy Intake Across the Day and Weight Loss: A Systematic Review and Meta-analysis," *Obesity Reviews*, vol. 24, no. 3 (December 18, 2022): e13537.

14. Winona Cochran and Abraham Tesser (2014). "The 'What the Hell' Effect: Some Effects of Goal Proximity and Goal Framing on Performance," in Leonard L. Martin and Abraham Tesser. *Striving and Feeling: Interactions Among Goals, Affect, and Self-regulation* (New York: Psychology Press, 2014): pp. 99–120.

15. Jaya Saxena. "Gone to Seed," Eater.com (June 10, 2025).

16. David Brooks. "Why Do So Many People Think Trump Is Good?" TheAtlantic.com (July 8, 2025).

17. Fariha Róisín. *Who Is Wellness For? An Examination of Wellness Culture and Who It Leaves Behind* (New York: HarperWave, 2022): chapter 3.

NOTES

Chapter 3: The Three Dead-Ends

Epigraph. Bono. "A Clenched Fist and an Open Hand: Lessons Learned from Desmond Tutu." Time.com (December 31, 2021).

1. "Overweight and Obesity Statistics," National Institute of Diabetes and Digestive and Kidney Diseases, niddk.nih.gov (accessed June 25, 2025).
2. "Type 2 Diabetes," Centers for Disease Control and Prevention, CDC.gov (May 15, 2024).
3. "Cardiovascular Diseases (CVDs)," World Health Organization, WHO.int (June 11, 2021).
4. As medical doctor Chris van Tulleken says in *Ultra-Processed People : Why We Can't Stop Eating Food That Isn't Food* (New York: W.W. Norton & Co., 2025): "Fix poverty, and you fix most diet-related diseases at the same time." The modern food system combined with harsh socioeconomic realities creates a huge barrier for public health.
5. Health Essentials (blog). "Why People Diet, Lose Weight and Gain It All Back," ClevelandClinic.org (October 1, 2019).
6. Jamie Rinaldi. "CPE Monthly: Effects of Chronic Dieting, Weight Fluctuations," *Today's Dietician*, vol. 26, no. 1 (January 2024).
7. Anna Guerdjikova. "Dangers of Dieting: Why Dieting Can Be Harmful," LindnerCenterofHOPE.org (February 8, 2024).
8. Jake Linardon, Tracy L. Tylka, and Matthew Fuller-Tyszkiewicz. "Intuitive Eating and Its Psychological Correlates: A Meta-analysis," *International Journal of Eating Disorders*, vol.54, no. 7 (March 30, 2021): pp. 1073–98. Also *see*, Tracy L. Tylka. "Development and Psychometric Evaluation of a Measure of Intuitive Eating," *Journal of Counseling Psychology*, vol. 53, no. 2 (April 1, 2006): pp. 226–40; and Kara N. Denny, Katie Loth, Marla E. Eisenberg, et al. "Intuitive Eating in Young

Adults: Who Is Doing It, and How Is It Related to Disordered Eating Behaviors?: *Appetite*, vol. 60, no. 1 (January 2013): pp.13–9.

9. Ashley N. Gearhardt, Sonja Yokum, Patrick T. Orr, et al. "Neural Correlates of Food Addiction," *Archives of General Psychiatry*, vol. 68, no. 8 (August 2011): pp. 808–16.

PART TWO

Chapter 4: Revealing Your Code

Epigraph. Don Richard Riso. *Enneagram Transformations: Releases and Affirmations* (New York: Houghton Mifflin Company, 1993): p. 3.

1. Becky Kennedy. Good Inside: A Guide to Becoming the Parent You Want to Be (New York: HarperCollins, 2022).

Chapter 5: Your Survival Eater

Epigraph. Ivan Pavlov. Nobel Lecture, Institute of Experimental Medicine, St. Petersburg, Russia (December 12, 1904).

1. I don't want to gloss over the fact that millions of American go hungry every day, including many children. According to USDA research, in 2023, 13.5 percent of U.S. households were food insecure at least some time during the year, meaning the households had difficulty providing enough food for all their members because of a lack of resources. "Food Security and Nutrition Assistance," Economic Research Service, U.S. Department of Agriculture website (updated July 24, 2025).

Chapter 6:Your Pleasure Eater

Epigraph. Robert Louis Stevenson. *An Inland Journey* (1878).

1. adrienne maree brown. *Pleasure Activism: The Politics of Feeling Good* (Chico, CA.: AK Press, 2019): p.13.

NOTES

Chapter 7: Your Social Eater

Epigraph. Patrice Apodaca. "Column: Blaze Bernstein's Memory also Lives on in the Kitchen," latimes.com (November 4, 2019).

1. Cesar E. Chavez Foundation. "Education of the Heart: Cesar Chavez in His Own Words," UFW.org/research (accessed June 21, 2023).
2. F. Luca, G.H. Perry, and A. Di Rienzo. "Evolutionary Adaptations to Dietary Changes." *Annual Review of Nutrition*, vol. 30 (August 21, 2010): pp,291–314.
3. Jan-Emmanuel De Neve, Andrew Dugan, Micah Kaats, et al. "Sharing Meals with Others: How Sharing Meals Supports Happiness and Social Connections," *World Happiness Report 2025* (accessed June 23, 2025).
4. Stefani J. Goldman, C. Peter Herman, and Janet Polivy. "Is the Effect of a Social Model on Eating Attenuated by Hunger?" *Appetite*, vol. 17, no.2 (October 1991): pp.129–40.
5. Nicholas A. Christakis and James H. Fowler. "The Spread of Obesity in a Large Social Network over 32 Years," *New England Journal of Medicine*, vol. 357, no. 4, (July 26, 2007): pp. 370–9.
6. De Neve, et al.

Chapter 8: Your Strategic Eater

Epigraph. Dwight D. Eisenhower. Remarks made at the National Defense Executive Reserve Conference on November 14, 1957. *Public Papers of the Presidents of the United States: Dwight D. Eisenhower, 1957* (Washington, D.C.: Federal Register Division, National Archives and Records Service, General Services Administration, 1934): p. 818.

Epigraph. Elliot T. Berkman, "The Neuroscience of Goals and Behavior Change," *Consulting Psychology Journal*, vol. 70, no. 1 (March 2018): pp. 28–44. Paul Rozin. "The Meaning of Food in

Our Lives: A Cross-cultural Perspective on Eating and Well-being," *Journal of Nutrition Education and Behavior*, vol. 37, supp. 2 (November–December 2005): pp. S107–12.

1. Paul Rozin. "The Meaning of Food in Our Lives: A Cross-cultural Perspective on Eating and Well-being," *Journal of Nutrition Education and Behavior*, vol. 37, supp. 2 (November–December 2005): pp. S107–12.

2. Lea Décarie-Spain, Cindy Gu, Logan, Tierno Lauer, et al. "Ventral Hippocampus Neurons Encode Meal-related Memory," *Nature Communications*, vol. 16 (June 11, 2025): article 4898.

3. Daniel Kahneman. *Thinking, Fast and Slow* (New York: Farrar, Straus and Giroux, 2011).

4. Wendell Berry. "The Pleasures of Eating," Ecoliteracy.org (June 29, 2009).

5. Rebecca Puhl. "Combating Weight Bias: Why We Need to Take Action," ObesityAction.org (summer 2017). Also *see*, Melody Fulton, Sriharsha Dadana, Vijay N. Srinivasan. *Obesity, Stigma, and Discrimination StatPearls* (Treasure Island, FL.: StatPearls Publishing [Internet], updated October 26, 2023).

6. Jean-Pierre Montani, Yves Schutz, and Abdul G. Dulloo. "Dieting and Weight Cycling as Risk Factors for Cardiometabolic Diseases: Who Is Really at Risk?" *Obesity Reviews*, vol. 16 (2015): pp. 7–18.

PART THREE

Chapter 9: Inner Leadership

Epigraph. Simon Sinek. *Start with Why: How Great Leaders Inspire Everyone to Take Action* (New York: Portfolio, 2009): p. 227.

1. When he said this to me, Able Cano was citing Marshall Ganz, Rita E. Hauser Senior Lecturer in Leadership, Organizing, and

Civil Society at the Kennedy School of Government at Harvard University.

2. Tara Brach. *Radical Acceptance: Embracing Your Life with the Heart of a Buddha* (New York: Bantam Dell, 2003): p. 44.

Chapter 10: Outer Mastery

Epigraph. John Little. *The Warrior Within: The Philosophies of Bruce Lee* (New York: Chartwell Books, 1996): p. 114.

1. Michael Pollan. *In Defense of Food: An Eater's Manifesto* (New York: Penguin Books, 2008): p.1.

Chapter 11: Making Peace with Food

Epigraph. David Peter Stroh. *Systems Thinking for Social Change: A Practical Guide to Solving Complex Problems, Avoiding Unintended Consequences, and Achieving Lasting Results* (White River Junction, VT.: Chelsea Green Publishing, 2015): p. 5.

Chapter 12: Eating in the Real World

Epigraph. Eduardo Galeano. *Walking Words*, translated by Mark Fried (New York: W.W. Norton & Co., 1997): p. 151.

RESOURCES
CONTINUE YOUR JOURNEY

Visit JeffSiegelWellness.com/wellness-plan-resources, or scan the QR code below, to access my **Wellness Resource Center**, where you'll find free courses, videos, and guides to help you create lasting change.

What you'll discover online:

- Commit to Sit 31-Day Learn to Meditate Course. This will help you build a daily practice step by step.

- Total Transformation Video Series. Four keys to aligning your past, present, and future for sustainable growth.

- Wellness Q&A offering practical answers to your biggest health and lifestyle questions.

- Articles and podcasts holding fresh insights on nutrition, fitness, mindfulness, and fatherhood.

- Guides and expert resources on topics from building a home gym to cultivating resilience and presence.

These tools are designed as a roadmap to better health—so you can take what you've learned here and put it into practice.

ABOUT THE AUTHOR

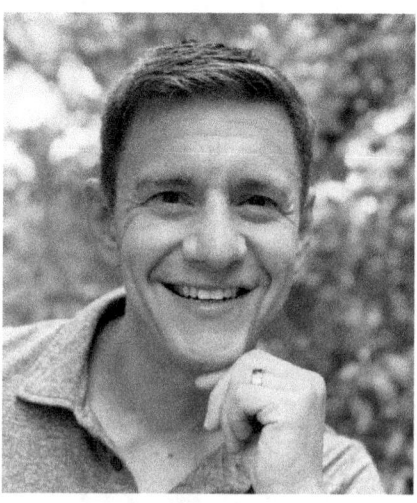

JEFF SIEGEL is a men's wellness coach, Harvard teaching fellow, and writer who empowers men to break free from destructive habits and thrive in today's complex food environment. Drawing on psychology, mindfulness, and nutrition science, his work helps men reconnect with their bodies and reclaim their health.

Jeff holds a master's degree in Mind, Brain, and Education from Harvard Graduate School of Education and a master's degree in Buddhist Studies from the University of Hong Kong. When he's not coaching or writing, you can find him biking around his home in Somerville, Massachusetts, or barefoot on beaches in New Jersey and Costa Rica, watching sunsets over the ocean with his wife and young son.

His debut book, *Eating 2.0*, introduces a system for eating well in an era of superabundance.

www.ingramcontent.com/pod-product-compliance
Lightning Source LLC
Chambersburg PA
CBHW060408130626
46555CB00005B/2002